Type 2 Diabetes Cookbook & Action Plan

I0134931

The Ultimate Beginner's Diabetic Diet Cookbook & Action Plan Guide to Reverse Pre-diabetes - Quick & Easy Delicious Healthy Type 2 Diabeic Recipes

By *Jennifer Louissa*

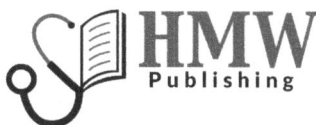

HMW Publishing

For more great books visit:

HMWPublishing.com

Get another book for Free

I want to thank you for purchasing this book and offer you another book (just as long and valuable as this book), "Health & Fitness Mistakes You Don't Know You're Making", completely free.

Visit the link below to signup and receive it:

www.hmwpublishing.com/gift

In this book, I will break down the most common health & fitness mistakes, you are probably committing right now, and I will reveal how you can easily get in the best shape of your life!

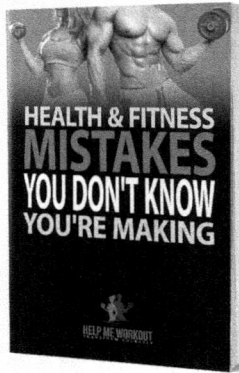

In addition to this valuable gift, you will also have an opportunity to get our new books for free, enter giveaways, and receive other valuable emails from me. Again, visit the link to sign up:

www.hmwpublishing.com/gift

Table of Contents

INTRODUCTION

Truth be told -- diabetes is tantamount to stories of struggles. And the very first struggle was to process the fact that you are in the pre-diabetic stage. It's never easy. The more you think about the disease, the more you get inundated with 'what if's'.

One reality that people living with diabetes need to deal with is how to come to terms with the disease on a daily basis. What to do? What not to do? What to eat? How not to suffer? And the list of questions continues. It can get pretty tiring at some point, especially when you are completely lost in the process.

But, one thing is certain -- you need to cultivate determination throughout the process. Yes, you need to stick your neck out and deal with it. You need to overcome your fear of this disease to be able to manage it.

Most importantly, you need an Action Plan.

In other words, you need that weapon to destruct

what could destruct you from the inside. Yes, an Action plan that entails your micro goals. Your ultimate goal is to reverse your pre-diabetes stage. Your micro goals, on the other hand, should direct your steps on how to strike a balance among your food, physical activities, and medication to combat the repercussions of this condition.

Bear in mind that diabetes is a lifelong disease. When you are unable to reverse the pre-diabetic stage, you will find yourself battling with a bigger monster. Love yourself more, and this book will help and guide you on how you can do this correctly. With the right action plan in hand, you will be able to take charge of your life.

Also, before you get started, I recommend you joining our email newsletter to receive updates on any upcoming new book releases or promotions. You can sign-up for free, and as a bonus, you will receive a free gift. Our *"Health & Fitness Mistakes You Don't Know You're Making"* book! This book has been written to demystify, expose the top do's and don'ts and to finally equip you with the information you need to get in the best shape of your life. Due to the overwhelming amount of mis-information and lies told by magazines and self-proclaimed "gurus", it's becoming harder and harder to get reliable information to get in shape. As opposed to having to go through dozens of biased, unreliable and un-trustworthy sources to get your health & fitness information. Everything you need to help you has been broken down in this book for you to easily follow and to immediately get results to achieve your desired fitness goals in the shortest amount of time.

Once again, to join our free email newsletter and to receive a free copy of this valuable book, please visit the link and signup now: www.hmwpublishing.com/gift

CHAPTER 1: THE TRUTH ABOUT DIABETES

WHAT DIABETES IS AND WHAT IT IS NOT?

What is diabetes - this is probably the very first question that crossed your mind when your doctor told you that you are in the 'pre-diabetic' stage. You have probably heard about the disease several times, but do not know what it is or how it develops.

When we eat, the food is processed and turns into glucose (sugar). Our body then uses the glucose as a source of energy. Our pancreas, on the other hand, produces insulin which enables the glucose to get into the cells of the body.

When you are diagnosed with diabetes or at the pre-diabetic stage, it could mean one of these two: either your body does not produce sufficient insulin or that your body is unable to use insulin well. When this happens, the glucose then builds up in your blood, and this when you develop diabetes.

Diabetes, by simple definition, means that your sugar level in the blood gets too high. Although your blood needs to have sugar in it to energize you, too much of it can be detrimental to your overall health. Specifically, it can damage several organs in your body including the kidneys, heart, eyes, and the nerves. The word itself pertains to the chronic disease that involves sugar levels and sweets which is why the next word you often see with *diabetes* is *mellitus.*

The word *Mellitus,* on the other hand, literally means sweet, sweetened, or honey – something along the line of sugary sweetness. The disease is officially called *Diabetes Mellitus,* but often, the medical world can do without including *mellitus* because everyone already knows what the word diabetes means and its general nature as a disease. So, to clarify any possible confusion in the future, *diabetes* and *diabetes mellitus* are the same.

ARE YOU AT RISK? CHECK THIS LIST!

Before we discuss the risk factors, let's have a quick glimpse at the two types of diabetes to understand better who are more prone to this disease.

Overall, there are two types of Diabetes, namely: Type 1 and Type 2. Another type is referred to as Gestational Diabetes which develops during pregnancy. About 1 out of 10 people inflicted with diabetes has Type 1 and is more common in children or younger adults. People with Type 1 diabetes tend to become dependent on injectable insulin as their pancreas can produce very little to no insulin at all.

The main reason behind this phenomenon is still unknown, and several types of research are on-going. This is to learn what prompts the body to attack the pancreas' beta cells and stop producing insulin. About 90% of people with diabetes suffer Type 2. In these cases, the pancreas produces insulin, but the body is not able to utilize the hormone very well. People with this condition discover about the case usually after the age of 30.

People who are likely to develop diabetes are those with the following conditions:

- A family history of diabetes

- Has a history of gestational diabetes

- Overweight or obese

Let's take a closer look at the different risk factors and what each of them means for the different types of diabetes. Take note of these and use the list for self-assessment.

RISK FACTORS FOR TYPE 1 DIABETES MELLITUS

While the principal cause of this disorder has not been identified yet, the factors that increase one's chance of developing it have been defined. These include the following:

History of the Family

This means that you have a higher chance of developing it if at least of your parents or siblings has it.

Dietary Factor and Eating Habits

Your choice of food plays a crucial role in the possible development of diabetes. Moreover, other related risk factors include minimal consumption of Vitamin D, early intake of cow's milk formula, and also the consumption of cereals before becoming four months old.

Environmental Factors

A person's exposure to specific viral illnesses may also trigger the development of this metabolic disease. The presence of auto-antibodies in your system. This is also referred to as a self-damaging immune system.

Geographic Factors

It has been found that people from some countries are more at risk of developing Type 1 Diabetes. These include Sweden and Finland.

RISK FACTORS FOR TYPE 2 DIABETES MELLITUS

Weight

Simply put, the more or thicker fatty tissues you have in your body, the more resistant you become to insulin.

Family History

As with Type 1, you are likely to develop diabetes if at least one of the immediate family members has diabetes.

Sedentary Lifestyle

In order words, being inactive -- physically inactive, for that matter, makes you even more prone to diabetes. This is because physical activity prompts your body to make use of glucose as your source of energy.

Age

Basically, the older you get, the more exposed you are to the risks of developing such disease. Reasons for this may include the change in your lifestyle as you tend to exercise less and consequently gain weight.

Race

One of the biggest mysteries behind diabetes is that individual races are more prone to it. These include Asian-Americans, Hispanics, American Africans, and Hispanics.

High Blood Pressure or Hypertension

Having a blood pressure that is over 140/80 millimeters of mercury is also associated with the risks of developing Diabetes as well.

Polycystic Ovarian Syndrome

This is a common condition that women with irregular menstruation, obesity, and excessive hair growth have. Those who are inflicted with this condition are also exposed to higher risks of developing diabetes.

Abnormal levels of triglyceride and cholesterol levels

If you high levels of 'bad' cholesterol and triglyceride, you are at risks of developing diabetes. This also means that your 'good' cholesterol or HDL is at a low level.

Gestational Diabetes

Women who had gestational diabetes while pregnant are also at risk of developing Type 2 later in life. Also, if you gave birth to relatively heavier babies (i.e., About 4 kilograms or above), you are also at risk.

HIGHLIGHTING FACTS AND

DISPELLING MYTHS

1. Keeping diabetes in check is as easy as 1, 2, 3

First things first, diabetes is not to be taken lightly. Just like cardiovascular disease that comes to you like a silent killer and then hits you without warning, diabetes is known for creeping up on you as well. And don't ever think that the worst is over after being diagnosed with diabetes. The worst is just about to start because being aware of it doesn't stop it from attacking you surprisingly again. So, no, it is never easy to keep diabetes in check.

2. Having diabetes means you'll have to have insulin shots

Well, that depends. If you are diagnosed with diabetes type 1 then, sadly, there is no other choice for you but to have insulin shots because it is

ALWAYS required. Now, if you have diabetes type 2, insulin shots are not needed every time. If your diabetes is controllable with some other medicines mainly to be taken orally, then there is no need for you to inject insulin. But, if not, then you will have to go for the injection method.

3. Sugar is the main culprit

While sugar is often INVOLVED when a person is diagnosed with diabetes, it does not mean that it is always the cause. Sometimes, it is just a contributing factor. The truth is, our bodies also require sugar. It does not only help us store energy, which is the function that gets messed up when a person has diabetes, but it is a vital part of our DNA or *deoxyribonucleic acid* – the primary material that carries all of our genetic information.

Also, diets that involve sugar also depend on the weight of the person consuming it. So if your diet is quite high in sugar, but you can maintain your average weight and insulin levels, you will not get diabetes because what many people think is "high" is actually what your body requires. However, if your weight is a little on the heavier side with a family history of diabetes, which is also a significant factor in being diagnosed with the disease, and your blood sugar is beyond reasonable then you should be a little careful with your sugar intake.

So, rejoice, people of the world! You can still enjoy sugar and sweets. Just make sure that you do not snack on it. To be sure, always see to it that you *include* them in your meals in proper servings or portioning.

4. Being overweight makes you an automatic diabetes type 2 patient

Not exactly. Let me sort it out for you. Being

overweight is a *serious risk* factor for developing diabetes type 2, yes. However it is just a *risk factor,* and it does not guarantee that you are, indeed, suffering from diabetes.

5. Obese or fat people are the only ones who get diabetes

This is so untrue. It is possible for thin people to develop diabetes as well if they are unable to control the levels of their blood sugar. Things only become worse especially if they have a family history of diabetes and it starts manifesting because of their ages, too. So, no. Just because you are fat does not mean you have diabetes and just because you are thin does not mean you are safe from having diabetes. Diabetes is way beyond *just the weight.*

6. Diabetes is incurable

That is what some doctors back then would say to you but, it is not entirely accurate. Diabetes *is only incurable* if you are not planning to change your lifestyle and diet. However, if you are willing to do anything just so you can live a couple more years to enjoy life with your loved ones, then definitely diabetes is curable. It is only a matter of discipline, priorities, diet, and lifestyle. I understand, it is easier said than done, but you have to start somewhere, right?

7. Diabetes is not serious

Okay, so we have settled the fact that diabetes is curable, but that does not mean it is not severe. **Diabetes is a chronic disease**, and if not appropriately managed or left unattended, it gets worse over time.

Now, before I get to the part where I emphasize the gravity of diabetes as a disease, let me explain the word *chronic* to give you a general feel of urgency when it comes to chronic diseases.

- Chronic – we hear this word from our doctors too often that we have learned just to ignore it and the message that it is trying to convey. For someone who has an inkling about the words *chronic disease*, they would think it merely pertains to a condition that has been ongoing for quite some time. This statement is true, *however,* only partly.

  Chronic disease pertains to the kind of illness that has been ongoing for quite some time in a very persistent manner. It causes long-term effects that may include complications that are altogether difficult to get rid of.

That being said, let us now return to the topic at hand – diabetes. Apart from the fact that it is chronic, diabetes in advance cases brings in its wake a myriad of complications such as kidney diseases, cardiovascular diseases *also known as heart diseases*, and other combo diseases that you would not want to worry yourself with anymore.

So, please, if you do not want to make it more complicated than it already is, do not take it lightly and act as soon as you can.

8. People with diabetes do not have insulin in their bodies

This is a baseless theory. Diabetes has two types, each with their characteristics.

Diabetes type 1 –

- Incapable of insulin production due to the immune system *incorrectly attacking* the pancreatic beta cells responsible for insulin production.

- Usually diagnosed while the patient is in his childhood.

- Does not often have something to do with being overweight.

- **Always** require insulin shots to control the disease.

- Often involves normal levels of ketone upon diagnosis.

Before we move on to the other type of diabetes, let us first talk about what *ketones* are.

- Ketones are molecules that are produced by the liver ***when*** a person is not eating correctly (*high sugar diet, excessive carbohydrate restriction, improper diet leading to starvation*), when doing an exercise that is too strenuous for long periods of time, and when suffering from insulin deficiency or diabetes type 1. Ketones are what comes after your body burns fat to keep you fueled.

What does it have to do with diabetes?

Since a diabetic's body does not produce insulin, which helps convert sugar into energy, glucose or sugar that is not converted enters your bloodstream. So, instead of joining the cells, glucose stays in the bloodstream coating your blood cells in the process and coats the insides of your arteries as well.

The results:

- Your blood becomes sugary sweet ***and thick*** *(This is why in advance cases of diabetes, you might see some patients being surrounded by ants, literally.)*

- Your arteries become narrower, or worse, clogged

- Thick blood + narrow arteries = high blood pressure **OR**

- Thick blood + clogged arteries = atherosclerosis (arteries becoming hard due to clogging formed by thick blood), **OR** an aneurysm (ruptured arteries due to blood not being able to pass through because of the clog), **OR** stroke.

Such a horrible equation, but it is the truth, and the explanation is far from being done.

Going back to the topic, our cells still needs something to burn so, burn they go. But, in the absence of glucose (*since glucose is busy doing nothing while staying in the bloodstream where they are not supposed to be in),* the next best thing that our cells choose to burn are fats. And so, ketones *or **acids*** are produced.

So, what?

Well, the body goes through **ketoacidosis**. Ketoacidosis is when your body produces too much acid that disturbs the body's natural pH.

What is pH?

pH is the unit of measurement of alkaline and acid in the body. The body's average pH level **should** stay between degrees of 7.30 to 7.45, meaning *slightly* alkalic. Anything below 7.30 level says your body is acidic or is undergoing ketoacidosis. Anything above 7.45 level means your body is too alkalic.

If a body goes through ketoacidosis and not treated immediately, it will lead to *diabetic coma* because the blood sugar is either too high (**hyper***glycemia)* or too low (**hypo***glycemia).* This state pushes the body and the blood sugar to extremes and if not immediately attended to, can lead to death.

Diabetes type 2 –

- Has insulin in the body, it's just that the body has developed resistance to it rendering the insulin useless.

- People in middle age are the ones often diagnosed with the disease.

- Being overweight plays a significant role in this disease.

- involves high levels of cholesterol and blood pressure

- in some cases, can be controlled with oral medications

- can be treated initially with proper lifestyle and diet

9. Being diagnosed with diabetes calls for dialysis

Renal disease or failure (*kidney disease or kidney failure*) is a complication of unmonitored diabetes. Meaning, if you take good care of yourself after being diagnosed with diabetes, monitor what needs monitoring and control what needs controlling so that you can avoid having to manage complications on top of diabetes.

10. Insulin takes care of it all

This is not true. Taking insulin, in the case of diabetes type 2, makes sure that you have the right amount of energy converted from sugar and then adequately utilized. It means your diet has to cooperate with your insulin intake to make sure that your body is not stuffing itself full of unused insulin and sugar that eventually gets mixed in your blood making it thicker, leading to advanced diabetes and even heart disease. If you do not change your diet and lifestyle, then don't be surprised if your diabetes gets worse faster than you can imagine.

11. Diabetes type 1 is worse than diabetes type 2

Being diagnosed with any of the two is bad enough. If you do not budge to keep your diabetes in control, whether it is type 1 or 2, it will finish you off like the silent killer it is – fast and without remorse.

12. Insulin causes blindness

Not true. Diabetes, if left unmonitored and uncontrolled, causes blindness. Ignorance is a complication of diabetes in its advanced stage, much like kidney failure and heart disease. If blindness occurred because a person used insulin, it's highly likely that the diabetes of that person has been ignored for quite a long time.

13. Diabetes is a pancreatic disorder

Diabetes is not a pancreatic disorder. It depends on the type of diabetes that you have, but if you have diabetes type 1, then what it is, is an *autoimmune disease*.

First, pancreatic disorder *or pancreatitis* is an inflammation of the pancreas. ***Any medical term that has a suffix of –itis pertains to inflammation.***

In the case of diabetes, the pancreas has long been inflamed and too severe to be even considered merely a pancreatic disorder. Fact is, pancreatic disorder leads to diabetes if left untreated. Think of it like this: **Acute Pancreatic Inflammation** (*acute, meaning short-term and abrupt onset of the disease*) is the seed, **Chronic Pancreatic Inflammation** is the seedling, and that one humongous monster tree is **Diabetes**.

How so? Like I mentioned awhile ago, in diabetes type 1, the immune system reacts incorrectly by attacking the pancreas leading to the inability of our body to produce insulin. As for diabetes type 2, it is considered a metabolic disorder, but research is being performed because the medical world is looking at the possibility of *autoimmune disease* angle

REVERSING PRE-DIABETES WITH NUTRITION. IS IT POSSIBLE?

To cut to the chase, yes it is possible. The earlier you learn about your condition, the better it is. To reverse pre-diabetes, you have to maintain a diet that is tailor-fit to you with the help of your doctor. Below is a general guideline for reversing pre-diabetes.

1. **Take it seriously.**

    Pre-diabetes is just a notch away from getting actual diabetes, and if you do not treat it correctly this time, chances are you will also have a problem with *practical* diabetes in the future. Do not wait for it to happen and be as precautious as you can. It might be a little confusing to adjust to this kind of lifestyle, but this is better than getting sick, right?

2. **Monitor your blood sugar at least 2-3 times a week.**

    Pre-diabetes patients shouldn't only stick to A1C tests. You should also make sure that you know what is happening to your blood sugar weekly. This is to help you find out if your current diet is helping or not.

Customize your diet with your doctor as soon as you can, to smoothly reverse pre-diabetes.

3. Watch what you eat.

You can still enjoy a cheat day despite being in this pre-diabetes state, but you have to be vigilant and disciplined for the rest of the week. You see, keeping your body in a healthier shape can help you a lot in reversing pre-diabetes. You do not need to be all toned and muscled. You merely need to keep the weight that is ideal for your body type, age, and gender. Doing this may also help you *off* from medications if your doctor already prescribes you some.

Opt for fishes and avoid sugar as much as you can, especially the processed ones. Sugar does not only cause you diabetes, but it also creates sluggishness. Also, make your skin look older if you have been bingeing on it. Your body will thank you for the excellent little gestures that you do.

4. Exercise

Lack of exercise will lead to weight gain and with weight gain on the horizon, the fight to reverse pre-diabetes will soon go out of the window. Weight gain expedites the possibility for you to get actual diabetes so make sure that you get at least a minimum of 15-minute a day exercise to combat this potential.

Exercise may seem like a chore to you, but many people with type 2 diabetes have sworn to this. A day of activity gives so much benefit for you to even pass up on the opportunity to do it while not busy. Your exercise does not need to be strenuous for you to reap its benefits. What matters is including it in your routine and following it religiously.

I know two people personally, one who swears on brisk walking for 30-45 minutes every day and the other one swears on playing table tennis for an hour twice a week. Both people mentioned were diagnosed to be pre-diabetic and are now well away from being actual diabetics. They also do not have to drown themselves on pre-diabetic medications too.

5. Notify your doctor of any changes you notice on your body

Anything strange that happens to your body must be reported to your doctor. Black or dark spots developing on areas you just scratched on, frequent urinating, wounds that are still fresh and getting infected even after two weeks – those are signs of a person with diabetes, and you have to make sure that your doctor knows if ever anything comes up. This is to help adjust your diet and prescribe you proper medications if needed.

I JUST FOUND OUT I HAVE DIABETES. WHAT DO I DO?

1. Do not panic.

I understand this is not an easy feat, considering you just found out that your life is in danger. However, you have to be composed. Do not even think of lingering or taking too much self-pity. It is not going to help you in any way. Keep your composure, cry or share your feelings and fears to a loved one, and slowly pull yourself together. You will need a focused mind and determination.

2. Health plan coverage.

While your frightened mind is thinking about many things, you will need, what you will feel and many other things that eventually lead to thinking about the unforeseen expenditures for your new-found condition, remind you that there is one thing that needs to be examined first – your health plan. Find out if it covers your condition or not. If included, what are the details? Does it cover medication or specialists? What are the restrictions? If not, find out what needs to be done. This way, you do not have to keep worrying about everything that has to do with your diabetes treatment. Your health plan will be able to provide you more time to worry and enjoy other things despite your new condition.

3. Diet

Before signing yourself up for any medication, feel free to go back to your physician and ask if you are still eligible to try reversing it by changing your diet. If yes, find out what kind of diet plans can suit you or better yet, they might be able to point you to the right direction of a good diabetes dietitian who knows the nitty-gritty details of the disease itself. This way, you get to tailor-fit your diet plan well.

If your condition is way past *just changing your diet plan,* then you may start considering medications. Do not forget to ask what each medicine is for if you are prescribed with more than one.

4. Exercise

Just because you found out you are sick, does not mean you have to stay in your room and feel depressed or suddenly make the significant change in your lifestyle. Take things a little slow. Of course, I will not ask you to take a pause and smell the flowers, but do not overwhelm yourself. Consider adding exercise to your daily routine because you cannot stay idle if that is how you have been before to being diagnosed. Being idle will only increase your risk of developing advanced diabetes.

Do what you enjoy best. If you are the gym kind of person, consider aerobic, flexibility, or resistance exercises. If not, feel free to enjoy dancing such as Zumba, recreational swimming, brisk walking, yoga, or even martial arts. Exercising does not need to be boring or too official. Keep it fun and incorporate it into your daily routine.

5. Socialize

Like I said earlier, do not welcome the negative emotions. The situation is already negative enough even to have room for the sad and scary things that your mind creates randomly. Your mind will keep doing that, it is wired to protect you so it will worry as much as it can, but do not swim in the emotions. Just take it to heart that yes, you got your mind's warning and then move on with your life. You are not yet dead, so live and be happy. Communicate with loved ones, communicate with those who have diabetes as well. Find and join a diabetic group if that is what you think you need, but never, ever welcome the negativity.

To feel sad for a while or even cry is just fine. But never go on for days feeling hopeless. This is not the way to live. Share ideas, tips, and even lifehacks with your diabetic community, surely they have some. This will make battling your condition a lot easier.

6. Supplies

After gathering helpful information from your diabetic community or friends who have experience with diabetes on their own or through a loved one, you may start supplying. Of course, you cannot go to a battle unarmed, so arm yourself with what is needed for your treatment.

One of the most common things that people with diabetes need is the blood glucose meter, lancing device, and test strips. You cannot do without them. Medications and other methods depend on the type of treatment you and your physician have talked about. Make sure consultation comes first before buying your supplies.

7. While at it, explore.

You may spend some time on finding out more about your condition. There is much information about it all over the internet; there are also books and even programs that can help you explore. Don't just stay in that one dark corner. Find out what you can about diabetes. Treat it like an enemy, find out what it is and find out its weakness. You will find the extra knowledge handy as you go on in life.

8. Schedule

If you are not the regular kind of person, you will severely need to plot a program that you must follow every day. One thing about diabetes is that it needs to be taken care of in a routine manner. Break that routine, and you might just find yourself wondering when your blood sugar started skyrocketing. Some people will just fall unconscious or crawl to get medical help if they stay clueless with their blood sugar levels for a day or two. Do not wait for this to happen to you.

Plot a schedule that includes your morning monitoring of blood sugar. This lets you determine how you will eat for the rest of the day. Include your medication schedule as well or insulin shots, if you are using this kind of treatment. You cannot forget these things. Set the alarm if you must.

9. Free time

Last, but not the least, never forget your free time. Again, you are sick, not yet dead. You deserve free time. It is good that you are starting to learn how to manage living while fighting diabetes, but every fighter needs to rest as well. Take a break, enjoy, recuperate, and then once you are well-rested, put your game face on and fight again.

Never forget to spare some free time for your family, loved ones, and yourself. This is what keeps you going, what keeps you sane. Spend quality time with people that love and understand you, enjoy your hobbies and other interests. You are still you; you did not change. It is just that you have to fight quite a big battle, but you should not let that struggle take your personality and dreams away.

Chapter 2: Living with Diabetes

The Diabetic's ABC

A1C

Surely you are familiar with the devices that help you monitor your blood sugar at home, right? They're handy, and they're fast. They do what is expected for it to do – to give you a reading where you can base your food intake or insulin dosage. However, these things are for just that, reading and insulin dosage. It doesn't give you any other details that can help physicians be precise with their treatment approach with your diabetes.

That's where A1C comes in. While your regular blood sugar monitor gives you the general status of your blood sugar, the A1C gives you the percentage of the blood cells in your body that is already wrapped in sugar. Yes, that is what happens to your blood if there's just too much sugar – it becomes your blood's coating. A1C doesn't only help monitor diabetes; it also helps those with prediabetes to know whether their condition is becoming better or worse.

It is to be performed three times a year if you are having a problem controlling your diabetes and twice a year to those who can manage their diabetes well.

Here is your guideline for A1C results:

Percentage	Translation of Blood Sugar Levels
5.7% or less	Normal
5.8 – 6.4%	Elevated / Prediabetes
6.5 % or more	Diabetes

BLOOD PRESSURE

As someone with diabetes, you've been monitoring your blood pressure, right? It's for monitoring purposes, so you'd know what is happening to your blood. But why do you want to know what is happening to your blood? What is it for?

Simple. As sugar coats your blood and it passes through your arteries, your arteries get their share of some sugar coating as well – but it happens INSIDE the arteries. In effect, your arteries become narrower, and you become at risk for heart attack and other heart diseases.

And so, what if your arteries becomes narrower, you may think? Think of your regular garden hose. Remember how when you want to play with water as a kid, you block the garden hose's end with your thumb? Then you proceed to open the faucet, so the water comes out of it faster to make that fun splash.

The same principle applies to your blood and arteries. The narrower the passage, the higher the pressure gets for it to pass through your arteries successfully. It's fun with water, but not with your blood. That is something you do not want happening to you. People die, garden hoses do not, and that is precisely why you are monitoring your blood sugar levels.

Blood Pressure	Translation of Blood Pressure
90/60 mmHg* or lower	Hypotension (Low blood pressure)
110/75 mmHg* – 120/80 mmHg*	Normal
120/80 mmHg* – 140/80 mmHg*	Early High Blood Pressure
140/90 mmHg* or higher	Hypertension (High blood pressure)

mmHg (millimeter of mercury) - *a unit of measurement used to determine the amount of pressure.*

Take note that the above indicated is the ideal blood pressure. While most people find it that their blood pressure translation matches easily with the chart above (as surely if you are experiencing hypotension or hypertension, your body WILL let you know), some people do not match this blood pressure translation too. In case your blood pressure translation doesn't match the chart (say for example, at 140/90 mmHg you still feel normal and absolutely no usual signs of hypertension), then I would suggest that you consult your doctor and find out YOUR healthy blood pressure levels. Blood pressure levels may vary with age, weight, lifestyle, and present conditions.

CHOLESTEROL

When you hear the word *cholesterol*, evidently you instantly think that it is terrible. Let me clarify it for you. Cholesterol is a part of your body, apart from the fact that it is also found in foods like dairy, meat, poultry, and seafood. It is an essential component that helps your body digest fat accurately, produce vitamin D, cell membranes, and hormones. Now, that's the right cholesterol you hear about.

There is also the lousy cholesterol also known as LDL or low-density lipoprotein. What does lousy cholesterol do to us?

For one, cholesterol is a substance made of fat. The sad part is that fat does not melt in water, and so, there is no way for it to travel our bloodstream on its own unlike other substances like sugar. Thus, our ever talented bodies thought of binding cholesterol or those fats to some proteins that can travel our bloodstream without any problem. Think of proteins like a cab inside our bodies that offers bloodstream transportation. So, in turn, the cholesterol that is bound to some of our proteins form a combination and **_LDL, or bad cholesterol is one of them_**.

Once your blood is found to contain a high percentage of this *bad cholesterol*, then it is a sure-fire sign that you are at risk of developing cardiovascular disease. Just imagine all those bad fats being transported and spread evenly to your whole body through your blood.

What do you need to do then? A fasting blood test and a proper diet. This enables you to identify your levels of cholesterol types HDL, LDL, and triglycerides.

You may refer to the chart found on the following page.

The chart contains the data or measurements that

is ideal for a person to keep themselves safe from developing diabetes or to prevent it from advancing.

LDL, HDL, and Triglycerides are measured separately. LDL will be measured, and it should not go over 100mg/dl. Anything over the given measurement means danger for you. As for HDL, the analysis should not be any lower than 50mg/dl, or it is heart disease for you. Lastly, with triglycerides, it should be at around 150mg/dl or lower. If it goes higher, you are in for a lifetime of heart disease.

Cholesterol Type	Proper Levels
LDL	100 mg/dl or lower
HDL	50 mg/dl - 70mg/dl or higher to avoid heart disease
Triglycerides	150 mg/dl or lower

__mg/dl__ - milligrams per deciliter. Used to measure glucose concentration in the blood.

GETTING ON WITH THE RIGHT NUTRITION

Seeing as there's just a lot of foods that hide under the bracket of LDL and sugar, how do you eat then? You're not supposed to starve yourself no matter what sickness you have and so, here's what you can eat to survive and enjoy life like you don't have diabetes at all.

1. **Dark, Green, Leafy Vegetables (Non-starchy)**

    Vegetables are low in carbs and have few calories, packed with fibers, vitamins, and has proteins as well. Fibers help your digestion, and proteins can give you *a part* of your required protein intake. This means you do not need to stuff yourself with meat every time anymore; you can go for the proper meat servings because of vegetables.

While most of us love meat, the truth is that it is harder to digest and there's also a big chance that it Is packed with cholesterol in between the meat strands if you were too lazy picking up your grocery. So, go for vegetables in the meantime that you are guilty *because the meat you have in the fridge **isn't** the lean type or worse, the processed type.*

2. Seafood

Seafood has proteins that are lean and are low in saturated fats. You need to avoid saturated fats at all costs. Enjoy 2-3 servings of fish, especially salmon, every week and you get to have the bonus of absorbing their omega-3 fats as well.

But, what is ***omega-3?***

Officially known as *Omega-3 fatty acids, these* are polyunsaturated fatty acids. By *polyunsaturated,* in layman's term, is the **healthier version of fat** that is good for the proper diet as compared to saturated fats.

There are three types of omega-3 fatty acids. One is called **DHA** or docosahexaenoic acid found in fatty fish oils, plant oils called ALA or a-linolenic acid, and the EPA or eicosapentaenoic acid/timnodonic acid also found in fatty fishes like salmon that lives in cold water.

Omega-3 fatty acids keep you safe from developing heart diseases by lowering triglyceride levels if it is elevated. Also, you get to have more benefits from it than just that, especially to those with asthma, depression, and arthritis. So, do not wait to get a result of a high triglyceride level. Enjoy your seafood and keep yourself healthy.

3. Whole Grains

Forget it if it does not have the word *whole* with it. You need entire grains because any grain that isn't whole is already processed and apart from the fact that the missing nutrients are replaced with sugar, who knows what else is in it? Whole grains help your digestion plus they keep you full longer. However, you have to be careful with the processed ones like your boxed cereals, pasta, white rice, and even the refined white flour.

4. Berries

Who doesn't like berries? Stuff yourself with these little things. They are packed with antioxidants, manganese, vitamin C, fiber, vitamin K, and potassium. Some of them are sweet, a little sour, but regardless they are all yummy and right for you.

5. Milk & Yogurt

An excellent source of calcium and most have been fortified to become a good source of Vitamin D; these things contain carbs that are good enough to fill in your daily needs as a person with diabetes. Just make sure to pick one that is low in sugar and fat.

6. Nuts

One ounce a day is what you need to keep your hunger at bay. They contain magnesium and fiber, and some even have omega-3 that is undoubtedly good for your heart.

7. Citruses

Citruses are excellent sources of folate, vitamin C, fiber, and potassium. They make your food zesty, and they fill out your daily vitamin requirements too.

8. Beans

Go for pinto, black beans, kidney beans, or

navy. They are stock full of minerals like potassium and magnesium, they are high in fiber and packed with vitamins too. Half a cup will do just fine for you to give you the right amount of goodies that you need without having to worry about the carbs they contain.

9. Tomatoes

We knew tomatoes are good for as even as a kid, so what changes that fact? Don't eat them cooked or you'll lose the good stuff. Have them raw to get the most out of the vitamins e and c and the potassium.

10. Stevia

This is not a part of superfoods, but feel free to enjoy it with your favorite drinks and foods. Stay away from sugar from now on and use stevia instead. It's all-natural and sweet. Have some fun with sweets without feeling guilty.

THE GLYCEMIC INDEX

Another important thing that you need to understand is the glycemic index, especially to those who take insulin. It shows you if there is a rise in your blood glucose levels after two hours that you have consumed a meal that has carbs in it. The measurement or ranking used for the glycemic index is from 0 to 100. Zero being the slowest food to raise your blood glucose levels and 100 being the fastest.

It mostly depends on the content of the food you eat, like the fats, carbohydrates, proteins, and even sodium.

It is used to help you and your doctor to find out how the food you eat reacts to your body and the insulin in it. Though, I have to make it clear that it is not used to measure your production of insulin even if your blood glucose levels rise. There is no *one size fits all* glycemic index. It varies for every food type and also takes note of the serving size and contents as factors to consider.

So, what is in it for you apart from helping you find out how your body reacts to the food you eat? The glycemic index can help you avoid sudden rise or *spike,* as many people call it, by identifying the foods that are ranked high. The higher glycemic index of the food, the more you should avoid it as it will raise your blood sugar levels in a flash.

Foods that get the glycemic index score of 70 or above is considered high in the index and are mostly composed of foods that are not good for you like processed foods, white bread, pizza, and many other store-bought foods. Foods that score 56 to 69 are considered medium like some fruits that *may* contain natural sugars, some healthier version of your usually unhealthy food like ice cream. The safest glycemic index scores are 55 and less. These include many vegetables like carrots, parsnips, yam, and green peas and fruits like pears, prunes, and apples. It also contains skim milk, whole grain bread, legumes, and beans.

WHAT ABOUT ALCOHOL?

Well, let me make this quick. To those who regularly consume alcohol, also to those who drink more than what their bodies can tolerate, alcohol is not a good idea for people with diabetes, regardless if it is type 1 or type 2. You would not want to dare because there is no such thing as *optimal consumption* for people with diabetes. There is an actual fix, but before we get to that, let me explain the dangers of alcohol consumption for people with diabetes.

The reminder "drink moderately" is not exactly going to cut it anymore for people with diabetes. There is a little exception, but still, it is not as good as it sounds before. You cannot merely drink moderately because doing so will highly likely lead your blood sugar levels to rise.

Remember how almost every alcoholic drinks

contain carbohydrates. High levels of carbs, if you do not already know, is highly dangerous for people with diabetes as carbohydrates can cause your blood sugar level to rise dramatically. Even if you say that the alcoholic drink contains 2 to 3 grams of carbs, several bottles will hurt your blood sugar, and you would not want that to happen.

As for heavy drinking, it is dangerous as well. If alcohol moderately raises your blood sugar significantly, heavy drinking, on the other hand, makes your blood sugar *plummet* **dramatically** into levels that you would not ever dream of going to especially to those who are battling type 1 diabetes.

Deficient blood sugar levels can kill you in minutes. I saw a person, who is battling pre-diabetes experience a superficial blood sugar level, crawl on the floor, covered in cold sweat, and does not even know if she would vomit first or take care of her seemingly uncontrollable bowel movement.

It is frightening to witness.

In such an occasion, the person ***must be*** given medical attention **as soon as possible;** there is no room for delay in any manner. A delay will lead to that person's death so fast you would not know what hit you.

Going back to the topic, avoid alcohol as much as you can, especially sweet wine and beer. Rum, gin, vodka, and whiskey are also some drinks to prevent as they lead to the massive drop in sugar levels.

You may enjoy liquor once in a while but avoid the mixers as they have tons of sugar in them. Also, make sure that the alcohol you intend to enjoy is carbohydrate-free. If you want to be extra safe, you may add seltzer or water to your drink as well. Wines are also excellent, especially for the heart, just make sure they are not sweetened. And as always, do not go wasted.Don't You Dare Forget About the Routine Care

Everyone has to have their daily routine, either that or you risk messing up your whole day including eating and sleeping patterns. That goes for people with diabetes too. Treat it like this, if your body has been aching some time and sending you pain signals, it is begging for you to take care of it better than before. And what better way to repay the vessel that enables you to enjoy life with your family than setting up a healthy routine for it?

1. **Monitor**

   Monitoring frequency depends on what your doctor tells you, but the best time to start is in the morning. This enables you how to plan your meals for the rest of the day and before you take your insulin shots if you are to have them. It seems quite a job in the first few weeks, but you'll warm up to it and realize its importance soon enough.

2. Manage

It is a bit like sailing, without a heading (monitoring your sugar), you pretty much do not know where to go. As soon as you're done with monitoring and are used to your blood sugar's fluctuations, then you can refine the diet that was initially prescribed to you. Do not be overwhelmed if you are asked to change your diet. It's all for you and as soon as you are familiar with it and its effects on your body, you can make some adjustments to customize it further for your needs with the help of your doctor.

3. Stick

Stick to your medications especially the schedule. They are there for a reason and not taking them, well, defeats just that very purpose. Missing one plan of medicine intake can undo your hard work of maintaining your diet. Don't let it happen. Might as well keep a pillbox and put a magnet on it, stick it in your fridge. That way, you do not forget it.

4. Exercise

When I say training, walking will do. You do not need to weight the heavy stuff just to make a point to your body that you are, in fact, trying to keep it in shape. Keeping in shape is only secondary, it's your heart that we are trying to protect her. Make sure it stays active, and you burn what needs burning while you walk and enjoy that time of the day when it is most convenient for you.

What Is the Right Treatment for You

You are not one to decide it on your own. Once you are diagnosed with diabetes, you can't go all DIY on it. I'm not saying either that you should be too dependent on your doctor. It needs collaboration to figure out what is truly good for you. Inform your doctor what your body shows you and what your body's reactions are to certain medications and food, your doctor decides the dosages and frequencies, and you agree to settle for the right treatment.

This doesn't stop the first time you get diagnosed. As your body adjusts to medications and copes with age, your body will respond to previous drugs it wasn't okay with before and stop responding to medications you are used to. So, adjustment, acceptance, and cooperation are the key.

DIET + EXERCISE

Diet AND exercise is one type of treatment for diabetics, especially if newly diagnosed and the status of diabetes is not that serious. However, for diet and exercise, you have to understand that one cannot go without the other, they always have to be together to fortify the protection that you build for your body by controlling what you put in it and how you maintain it. Also, dieting for your diabetes should be tailor-fit for your needs. It's not like a ready-made t-shirt that you can just grab from a stand and try on. YOUR DIET SHOULD ALWAYS GO WITH YOUR AGE, WEIGHT, LIFESTYLE, and CURRENT CONDITIONS – no more, no less.

As for exercise, there's no need for you to go all out on it primarily if you are not used to strenuous activities. Walking or brisk walking with your loved one and your dog, doing yoga or your favorite martial arts, and even recreational swimming will do. Just make sure to do it every day for about 30, minutes, and you will do just fine.

ORAL MEDICATION

Oral Medication is the option when diet and exercise are not cutting it for you anymore. Some of these medications are to encourage your liver not to dispose of all the glucose that passes through it, some are meant to help prevent your pancreas from breaking down the hormones that help produce insulin, and some encourage your pancreas to produce more insulin.

There are many other medications for diabetes that will help you out directly, however, again this needs the go signal of your doctor if you are to start any of these medicines.

INJECTABLES

Just because you see a diabetic injecting medication does not mean it is already insulin. It's not always insulin. At times, there are medications that people with diabetes need to help them slow down their digestion. To prevent them from frequently eating to improve their livers by slowing down the glucose production. Just like oral medication, there is a myriad of function for injectable medicines meant for people with diabetes. Again, this depends on your doctor's findings and suggestions.

INSULIN

Not all diabetics need insulin injections or pumps. Those people with diabetes type 1 need insulin, but not always for those with diabetes type 2. Insulin is to be taken ONLY if your blood sugar is getting more and more difficult to control. There are other methods to get insulin into your body, and that is through injection, inhaler, through insulin pen, and even insulin pumps.

WEIGHT LOSS SURGERY

If none of the above is cutting it anymore for you and your doctor thinks that in your current state, having a weight loss surgery is the best option, then go for it. Please be advised that weight loss surgery is not for everyone and some people have to make do with the above options.

Weight loss surgery will, like the name says, a slash of a right amount of your weight and make controlling of your blood sugar a lot easier than it did before. As an effect, it increases the hormones *incretins* responsible for your pancreas' insulin production. It has a lot of benefits. But do not opt for this if your diabetes is still controllable with a combination of the above treatments unless you are overweight and your blood sugar is really out of control.

CHAPTER 3: CREATING A LIFE-CHANGING ACTION PLAN

Know Your Treatment Goals

What do you think is your ultimate treatment goal? Yes, that is to keep your blood sugar ALWAYS, ALWAYS, at bay. However, that is not as easy as you can say it. And so, you have to know it, remember it, and live with it.

Another thing that you have to add to your goal is to prevent tissue damage from happening to you because of too much sugar that flows into your bloodstream.

Since you already know your targets for healthy blood sugar by basing on the previous chapter, all you have to do is not to forget monitoring your blood sugar. When your schedule for an A1C test arrives, do not, AT ALL COST, skip it. Treat it as something significant because getting the results from that analysis will let you know if there have been good or bad changes in your diabetes. Surely, you do not want to keep to a diet that does not fit you anymore, right?

IDENTIFYING THE STEPS TO TAKE

The following are your regular *must-do*, every time you visit your doctor.

1. Monitor Your Blood Glucose

I know you have repeatedly been told to monitor your blood glucose so you'd know how to work on it as your day pans out. And I am repeating it now because your life depends on it, no kidding. So, wherever you go, may it be your house or the hospital, don't ever miss it.

2. Get Your Blood Pressure Monitored

The next most important thing after your blood sugar is your blood pressure. If you keep monitoring one without the other, then the purpose of your treatment is lost. Blood sugar and blood pressure go hand in hand because it involves both your blood and heart.

3. Check Your Foot

What's the foot got to do with your diabetes? Well, your feet are like the window to your diabetic body. Anything that goes exceptionally wrong with your blood circulation and even damage to your nerves will inevitably show through your feet. The same principle applies to diabetes and infections.

4. Check Your Weight

Your weight, apart from your feet, says a lot about your diet. It's not always an identifier of diabetes, *but* checking your blood glucose as soon as your weight rises is the best way of protecting yourself not only from diabetes but also heart diseases.

5. Review Your Treatment Plan

Always, always review your treatment plan with your doctor before you leave the hospital. You need to let your doctor know of any changes in your body's reaction to your current medication and diet as this *may* mean having to change your doses, medicine, and even your dietary plan.

6. A1C Test

Don't forget your A1C test as well. This analysis should be performed twice to thrice a year depending on the levels of your diabetes.

TRACKING YOUR PROGRESS

Why should you track your progress? Tracking your progress can help your physician more than you can imagine as your journal will contain details of your daily life as you try your best (and sometimes failing) to control your blood sugar and your diabetes in general.

Make sure to track:

- Weight gain

- Weight losses

- Eating habits

- Eating behaviours

- Daily blood sugar results

Be as honest as you can and do not ever think that you are doing it for your doctor. You are doing it for yourself to help you become better and to be successful in fighting your diabetes. If you are not as comfortable using a physical journal, there are numerous apps found on the internet that is made for diabetes alone. However, the problem with keeping your progress through an app is your battery's availability.

Still, go for one which makes you feel most comfortable. After all, the most important thing here is what can be found in your diabetes journal.

CHAPTER 4: THE HEALING DIET

To help you out with your battle with diabetes, let us not only stick with words of advice, steps to follow, tips, and encouragements. Let me spare a whole chapter for some yummy recipes that won't make you worry about your blood sugar.

7 SMOOTHIE RECIPE

RASPBERRY AND PEANUT BUTTER SMOOTHIE

Serves: 2

Preparation: 10 minutes

Ingredients:

- Peanut butter, smooth and natural [2 tbsp]
- Skim milk [2 tbsp]
- Raspberries, fresh [1 or 1 ½ cups]
- Ice cubes [1 cup]
- Stevia [2 tsp]

Directions:

Put in all the ingredients in your blender. Set the mixer to puree, wait until smooth. Serve. Good for 2.

Calories	Fat	Carbs	Protein	Sodium
170	8.6g	20g	5.1g	67mg

Strawberry, Kale and Ginger Smoothie

Serves: 2

Preparation: 10 minutes

Ingredients:

- Curly kale leaves, fresh and large with stems removed [6 pcs]
- Grated ginger, raw and peeled [2 tsp]
- Water, cold [½ cup]
- Lime juice [3 tbsp]
- Honey [2 tsp]
- Strawberries, fresh and trimmed [1 or 1 ½ cups]
- Ice cubes [1 cup]

Directions:

Put in all the ingredients in your blender. Set the mixer to puree, wait until smooth. Serve. Good for 2.

Calories	Fat	Carbohydrates	Protein	Sodium
205	2.9g	42.4g	4.2g	0.083 mg

ALMOND + BLUEBERRY SMOOTHIE

Serves: 2

Preparation: 10 minutes

Ingredients:

- Almonds, slivered [1/4 cup]

- Stevia [2 tsp]

- Wheat germ [2 tbsp]

- Blueberries, fresh [1 or 1 ½ cups]

- Greek yogurt [½ cup]

- Ice cube [1 cup]

- Almond or skim milk, unsweetened [2 tbsp]

Directions:

Put in all the ingredients in your blender. Set the mixer to puree, wait until smooth. Serve. Good for 2.

Calories	Fat	Carbohydrates	Protein	Sodium
225	8g	31g	11.4g	34mg

Cottage Cheese and Spiced Raspberry Smoothie

Serves: 2

Preparation: 10 minutes

Ingredients:

- Rolled oats, old-fashioned [2 tbsp]

- Cottage cheese, fat-free [½ cup]

- Dates pitted [2 pcs.]

- Stevia [1 tsp]

- Ice cubes [1 cup]

- Cinnamon, ground [1 pinch]

- Fresh raspberries, [1 ½ cups]

Directions:

Put in all the ingredients in your blender. Set the blender to puree, wait until smooth. Serve. Good for 2.

Calories	Fat	Carbohydrates	Protein	Sodium
134	1g	25g	8.4g	216mg

Flax Seed and Strawberry-Banana Smoothie

Serves: 2

Preparation: 10 minutes

Ingredients:

- Stevia [2 tsp]

- Skim milk [2 tbsp]

- Flaxseed, ground [2 tbsp]

- Tofu, soft [½ cup]

- Banana, medium-sized [sliced]

- Ice cubes [1 cup]

- Strawberries, fresh and trimmed [1 or 1 ½ cups]

Directions:

Put in all the ingredients in your blender. Set the blender to puree, wait until smooth. Serve. Good for 2.

Calories	Fat	Carbohydrates	Protein	Sodium
159	4.7g	25g	7.7g	10mg

Green Apple and Spinach Smoothie

Serves: 2

Preparation: 10 minutes

Ingredients:

- Stevia [2 tsp]

- Ice cube [1 cup]

- Greek yogurt [½ cup]

- Apple or orange juice, unsweetened [1/3 cup]

- Small apple, chopped and cored [1 pc]

- Stevia [1 tsp]

- Flax seeds. Ground [2 tbsp]

- Baby Spinach [2 cups]

Directions:

Put in all the ingredients in your blender. Set the blender to puree, wait until smooth. Serve. Good for 2.

Calories	Fat	Carbohydrates	Protein	Sodium
138	2.4g	24g	7.4g	69mg

BLACKBERRY AND NUTS SMOOTHIE

Serves: 2

Preparation: 10 minutes

Ingredients:

- Stevia [2 tsp]

- Greek yogurt [½ cup]

- Ice cubes [1 cup]

- Almond butter [2 tbsp]

- Blackberries, fresh [1 or ½ cup]

Directions:

Put in all the ingredients in your blender. Set the blender to puree, wait until smooth. Serve. Good for 2.

Calories	Fat	Carbohydrates	Protein	Sodium
175	9.3g	16g	9.6g	57mg

GREEN SMOOTHIES

GREEN DIABETIC SMOOTHIE

Serves: 2

Preparation: 10 minutes

Ingredients:

- Orange, large [1 pc]

- Kale [1 cup]

- Spinach [2 cups]

- Celery [3 stalks]

- Cucumber, large [1 pc]

- Ice cubes [1 cup]

Directions:

Put in all the ingredients in your blender. Set the blender to puree, wait until smooth. Serve. Good for 2.

Calories	Fat	Carbohydrates	Protein	Sodium
250	1g	30g	8g	0mg

DELECTABLE SWEET POTATO

SMOOTHIE

Serves: 2

Preparation: 10 minutes

Ingredients:

- Orange, large [1 pc]

- Sweet potato, cooked and peeled [½ cup]

- Banana, frozen [½ cup]

- Cinnamon [¼ tsp]

- Almond milk, unsweetened [1/2 cup]

- Almond butter [1 tbsp]

Directions:

Put in all the ingredients in your blender. Set the blender to puree, wait until smooth. Enjoy.

Calories	Fat	Carbohydrates	Protein	Sodium
262.5	4.9g	50.4g	4.6g	417.6mg

VERY BERRY SMOOTHIE

Serves: 2

Preparation: 10 minutes

Ingredients:

- Kale [3 pcs]
- Mango chunks, fresh [a handful]
- Blueberries, frozen [1 cup]
- Flax meal [2 tbsp]
- Blackberries, frozen [1 cup]
- Pure coconut water, unsweetened [2 cups]

Directions:

Put in all the ingredients in your blender. Set the blender to puree, wait until smooth. Enjoy.

Calories	Fat	Carbohydrates	Protein	Sodium
148	0g	35g	2g	25mg

GREEN, GREEN, GREEN

Serves: 2

Preparation: 10 minutes

Ingredients:

- Ginger, peeled and sliced [1 cm]

- Celery, cut into chunks [½ stick]

- Mint leaves [12 pcs]

- Cucumber, cut into thick slices [2 inches]

- Baby spinach [a handful]

- Cold press apple juice [1 ¼ cup]

Directions:

Put in all the ingredients in your blender. Set the blender to puree, wait until smooth. Enjoy.

Calories	Fat	Carbohydrates	Protein	Sodium
250	1g	33.4g	8g	0mg

Spinach, Chia Seed, and Coco Smoothie

Serves: 2

Preparation: 10 minutes

Ingredients:

- Ginger, peeled and sliced [1 cm]
- Celery, cut into chunks [½ stick]
- Mint leaves [12 pcs]
- Cucumber, cut into thick slices [2 inches]
- Baby spinach [a handful]
- Cold press apple juice [1 ¼ cup]

Directions:

Put in all the ingredients in your blender. Set the blender to puree, wait until smooth. Enjoy.

Calories	Fat	Carbohydrates	Protein	Sodium
354	4g	58g	22g	0.083 mg

Go Nutty-Berry Smoothie

Serves: 2

Preparation: 10 minutes

Ingredients:

- Ginger, peeled and sliced [1 cm]

- Chia seeds [2 tsp]

- Cinnamon [½ tsp]

- Almond butter [1 tbsp]

- Banana, frozen [½ a piece]

- Mixed berries, frozen [½ cup]

- Stevia [1 tsp]

- Almond milk [1 cup]

- Flaxseed, ground [1 tbsp]

Directions:

Put in all the ingredients in your blender. Set the blender to puree, wait until smooth. Enjoy.

Calories	Fat	Carbohydrates	Protein	Sodium
154.6	7.7g	21.3g	3.2g	91.6mg

YUMMY OATMEAL BERRY SMOOTHIE

Serves: 2

Preparation: 10 minutes

Ingredients:

- Old fashioned rolled oats [½ cup]

- Vanilla yogurt or Greek yogurt [⅓ cup]

- Frozen berries [½ cup]

- Ice cube [1 cup]

- Milk [1 cup]

- Stevia [2 tbsp]

Directions:

Put in all the ingredients in your blender. Set the blender to puree, wait until smooth. Enjoy.

Calories	Fat	Carbohydrates	Protein	Sodium
177	1g	32g	11g	20mg

7 - Chicken Recipes Ideal for Lunch and Dinner

Chicken Parmesan Drumstick: Finger-Licking Good Without the Guilt

Serves: 3-4

Ingredients:

- Paprika [1 tsp]

- Dried oregano, crushed [2 tsp]

- Lemon wedges

- Eggs, beaten [2 pcs]

- Black pepper [¼ tsp]

- Butter melted [¼ cup]

- Snipped fresh oregano

- Fine dry bread crumbs [¾ cup]

- Grated Parmesan cheese [¾ cup]

- Chicken drumsticks skinned [16 pcs]

- Fat-free milk [¼ cup]

Directions:

Set oven to 375 deg. F. Line, foil, and grease two shallow and large baking pans. Set aside. Combine egg and milk in a small bowl. In another shallow dish, add bread crumbs, paprika, oregano, parmesan, and pepper. Dip the drumsticks into the egg mixture and then coat with the crumbs. Place drumsticks in pans and drizzle with butter. Bake for 45 – 50 mins while uncovered. Wait for the chicken to become tender. Sprinkle with oregano and add lemon wedges for garnishing.

Calories	Fat	Carbohydrates	Protein	Sodium
336	4g	38g	38g	532mg

BUFFALO-STYLE CHICKEN SALAD: A HINT OF SPICE TO TICKLE YOUR PALATE

Serves: 2

Ingredients:

- Paprika [1 tsp]

- Fat-free blue cheese salad dressing [1 tbsp]

- Cracked black pepper [1/4 tsp]

- Cooked chicken breast, chopped [3/4 cup]

- Fat-free milk [1 tsp]

- Celery, cut into sticks [1 pc]

- Buffalo wing sauce [2 tbsp]

- Light blue cheese, crumbled

- Heart of romaine sliced [Half]

Directions:

Place the romaine in a bowl. Place chopped chicken and sauce in a microwave-safe bowl. Microwave the diced chicken and sauce on high for a minute. Add the microwaved mixture over the romaine. Add cheese and pepper for toppings. Combine milk and salad dressing and then drizzle over your salad. Add celery sticks and serve.

Calories	Fat	Carbohydrates	Protein	Sodium
297	10g	13g	37g	596mg

Louisiana Chicken: The Ultimate Companion for your Day or Night Meal

Serves: 2-3

Ingredients:

- Frozen cut okra [1 cup]
- Black pepper [1 tsp]
- Stewed tomatoes, no salt [1 can]
- Skinned drumsticks [8 pcs]
- Louisiana hot sauce [1 ½ tbsp.]
- Whole grain noodles, cooked [2 cups]
- Dried thyme, ground [1 tsp]
- Salt [1/4 tsp]

Directions:

Coat a skillet lightly with cooking spray. Place it over medium-high heat and add chicken. Let it turn brown on all sides and don't forget to set them. Add stewed tomatoes on top, thyme, hot sauce, okra, pepper, and salt. Let it boil and then reduce the heat. Cover and then simmer until the center is no longer pink. Add the chicken on a platter and then the sauce. Serve with the noodles and enjoy.

Calories	Fat	Carbohydrates	Protein	Sodium
190	1g	8g	27g	500mg

THAI CHICKEN WINGS: A QUICK FIX FOR YOUR EXOTIC DISH CRAVING

Serves: 7-8

Ingredients:

- Lime juice [1 tbsp]
- Ground ginger [1/4 tsp]
- Peanut Sauce
- Chicken wing drummettes [24 pcs]
- Water [1/4 cup]
- Crushed red pepper [1/4 tsp]
- Garlic, minced [2 cloves]
- Water [1/2 cup]
- Reduced-sodium soy sauce [2 tsp]
- Almond butter [1/2 cup]
- Ground ginger [1/2 tsp]

Directions:

Put chicken in the slow cooker. Add the lime juice, water, and ginger. Cover and set to low heat. Let it cook for 5-6 hrs. Drain the chicken and discard the liquid. Add half of the peanut sauce to chicken and toss. Serve.

Calories	Fat	Carbohydrates	Protein	Sodium
101	1g	3g	9g	159mg

CHICKEN MAC & CHEESE: DIABETIC-FRIENDLY AND JUST SUPER YUMMY

Serves: 2

Ingredients:

- Finely chopped onion [1/4 cup]
- Dried multigrain [1 ½ cups]
- Fresh baby spinach [2 cups]
- Skinless, boneless chicken breast halves, cut into 1-inch pieces [12 oz]
- Fat-free milk [1 2/3 cups]
- Chopped, seeded tomatoes [1 cup]
- All-purpose flour [1 tbsp]
- Shredded reduced-fat cheddar cheese [3/4 cup]
- Light semi soft cheese with garlic and herb [[1 6 1/2 oz]

Directions:

Cook the macaroni in a saucepan. Make sure to follow package directions. Don't add salt. Drain the macaroni. Coat a skillet with cooking spray. Heat the skillet over medium-high heat. Add the chicken and onions. Let it cook until onion is transparent and chicken is no longer pink. Stir frequently. Remove the skillet from heat. Add the cheese until it melts. Whisk flour and milk in another bowl. Add the chicken mixture. Cook over medium-high heat and stir. Wait until thick and bubbly then reduce the heat to low. Add the macaroni until heated. Add tomatoes and spinach. Serve.

Calories	Fat	Carbohydrates	Protein	Sodium
169	3g	24g	11g	210mg

Five Spice Chicken Wings: Put Your Fingers and

Serves: 4-5

Ingredients:

- Finely chopped onion [1/4 cup]

- Plum sauce [3/4 cup]

- Five-spice powder [1 tsp]

- Butter melted [1 tbsp]

- Slivered green onions

- Chicken wings [16 pcs]

Directions:

Preheat your oven to 375 deg. F. Cut off the tips of the wings and discard the tips. Cut each wing into two pieces. Line a baking pan with foil and arrange the wings in it in a single layer. Bake the wings for 20 minutes. Drain. In a slow cooker, add the butter, five spice powder, plum sauce and chicken. Stir to coat the chicken with sauce. Cover and cook on low heat. Do this for

4 hours. Serve.

Calories	Fat	Carbohydrates	Protein	Sodium
32	1g	3g	3g	45mg

Balsamic and Dijon Chicken: Your Ultimate Grilled Chicken Craving Buster

Serves: 2

Ingredients:

- Balsamic vinegar [3 tbsp]
- Snipped fresh thyme [2 tsp]
- Dijon-style mustard [1/3 cup]
- Garlic, minced [2 cloves]
- Skinless, boneless chicken breast halves [4 pcs]
- Fresh thyme sprigs

Directions:

In a resealable plastic bag placed over a shallow dish, add the chicken and set aside. Prepare the marinade by stirring the balsamic vinegar, mustard, thyme, and garlic until smooth. Pour the marinade on the chicken inside the plastic and seal the bag. Turn bag to coat the chicken and leave in the fridge for 24 hours. Turn the bag if needed. Drain the chicken, don't discard the marinade. Place the chicken on the grill directly over coals. Grill, the chicken for 7 minutes and brush with marinade. Turn the chicken and coat again with marinade. Garnish with thyme sprigs. Serve.

Calories	Fat	Carbohydrates	Protein	Sodium
161	1g	3g	26g	537mg

7 - Pork Recipes Ideal for Lunch and Dinner

Quick Pork Diane: Delectable Dish Under 30 Minutes

Serves: 4

Ingredients:

- Lemon juice [1 tsp]

- Snipped fresh chives, parsley, or oregano [1 tbsp]

- Water [1 tbsp]

- Dijon-style mustard [1 tsp]

- Butter [1 tbsp]

- Worcestershire sauce [1 tbsp]

- Lemon-pepper seasoning [1 tsp]

- Four boneless pork top loin chops

Directions:

To make the sauce, add water, lemon juice, mustard, and Worcestershire sauce in a bowl and set aside. Remove the fat from the chops and sprinkle each side with lemon-pepper seasoning. Melt butter in a skillet and add the chops. Cook for 12 minutes and turn to cook the other side. Remove from heat. Transfer to serving platter and cover with foil. Pour the sauce into the skillet and then pour the sauce over the chops. Top the chops with chives. Serve.

Calories	Fat	Carbohydrates	Protein	Sodium
178	11g	1g	18g	302mg

Mediterranean Pork Chops: A 5-Ingredient Dish You Wouldn't Want to Miss

Serves: 1

Ingredients:

- Boneless or bone-in pork loin chops cut 1/2 inch thick (1 pc)
- Salt [1/4 tsp]
- Freshly ground black pepper [1/4 tsp]
- Finely snipped fresh rosemary or 1 tsp dried rosemary, crushed [1 tbsp]
- Garlic, minced [3 cloves]

Directions:

Prepare the oven by preheating to 425 deg. F. Line a roasting pan with foil and sprinkle the chops with salt and pepper. Set aside. Add rosemary and garlic, combine in a bowl. Sprinkle them evenly on the chops. Place the chops in the pan. Roast for 10 minutes. Reduce the oven temp to 350 deg. F and serve.

Calories	Fat	Carbohydrates	Protein	Sodium
161	5g	1g	25g	192mg

Serves: 3-4

Ingredients:

- Sliced mango or chili peppers

- Lime juice [¼ cup]

- Olive oil [1 tbsp]

- Salt [¼ tsp]

- Garlic, minced [2 cloves]

- Ground cinnamon [1 tsp]

- Chili powder [1 tbsp]

- Ground cumin [2 tsp]

- Hot pepper sauce [½ tsp]

- Four pork rib chops, cut ¾ inch thick

Directions:

Place the chops in a plastic bag. To make the marinade, add chili powder, lime juice, cumin, oil, cinnamon, garlic, hot pepper, and salt. Pour them over the chops and seal the bag. Turn the bag to coat chops well. Place the chops in the fridge for 24 hours. Make sure to turn the bag to even out the marinade. Drain the chops and discard the marinade. Grill the chops until pork juices run clear. Turn once. Garnish with mango or chili peppers. Serve.

Calories	Fat	Carbohydrates	Protein	Sodium
196	9g	3g	25g	159mg

Tender Pork in Mushroom Sauce: That Perfect Comfort Dish For Every Occasion

Serves: 4

Ingredients:

- Cooking oil [1 tbsp]

- Worcestershire sauce [1½ tsp]

- Dried thyme, crushed [¾ tsp]

- 1 (10.75 ounces) can reduced-fat, reduced-sodium condensed cream of mushroom soup

- Pork loin chops, cut ¾ inch thick (4 pcs)

- Garlic powder [1 tsp]

- Apple juice or apple cider [½ cup]

- One small onion, thinly sliced

- Sliced fresh mushrooms [1½ cups]

- Fresh thyme sprigs

- Quick-cooking tapioca [2 tbsp]

Directions:

Remove the fat from the chops. Place a skillet over medium heat and add oil then warm. Add the chops and cook until brown. Drain the fat. Add the onion in a slow cooker and add the chops. Crush the tapioca and add it to a bowl together with Worcestershire sauce, thyme, garlic powder, apple juice, mushrooms and mushroom soup. Pour the mixture over the chops. Cover the slow cooker and cook on low heat for 8 to 9 hours. Garnished with thyme sprigs. Serve.

Calories	Fat	Carbohydrates	Protein	Sodium
152	2g	4g	26g	286mg

PORK AND HERB-TOMATO SAUCE: A SLOW-COOKED DISH PERFECT FOR THE FAMILY

Serves: 4

Ingredients:

- Quick-cooking tapioca crushed [2 tsp]

- Salt [¼ tsp]

- Worcestershire sauce [½ tsp]

- Minced garlic (3 cloves)

- Four pork rib chops (with bone), cut ¾ inch thick

- Small onion, chopped [1 pc]

- Stewed tomatoes, undrained and unsalted [2 cans]

- Crushed red pepper [1/4 tsp]

- Ground black pepper [½ tsp]

- Dried Italian seasoning, crushed [1 tsp]

Directions:

Remove the fat from the chops and lightly coat the skillet with cooking spray. Place skillet over medium-high heat. Cook the chops until brown on both sides and set aside. In a slow cooker, add the garlic, onion, tapioca, black pepper, Italian seasoning, crushed red pepper, Worcestershire sauce, and salt. Add the chops and pour the tomatoes. Cover the slow cooker and cook on low heat for 8 hours. Transfer the chops to a platter, add tomatoes on top and serve.

Calories	Fat	Carbohydrates	Protein	Sodium
245	7g	19g	24g	568mg

CRANBERRY PORK LOIN: SWEET AND TANGY, PERFECT FOR THE TUMMY

Serves: 4

Ingredients:

- Cooking oil [1 tbsp]

- Honey [1 tbsp]

- Salt [1/8 tsp]

- Ground nutmeg [1/8 tsp]

- Ground black pepper [1/8 tsp]

- Frozen orange juice concentrate, thawed [2 tbsp]

- Ground ginger [¼ tsp]

- Whole cranberry sauce [½ cup]

- 4 (5 ounces) boneless pork loin chops, cut ½-inch thick

Directions:

Coat a skillet with nonstick cooking spray and place over medium-high heat. Sprinkle salt and pepper on both sides of chops and put it on the skillet. Reduce the heat to medium and let the chops cook until done. Make sure you turn the chops. Remove the chops from the skillet and cover with foil. Add orange juice concentrate, honey, nutmeg, ginger, and cranberry sauce in a bowl and mix. Add the mixture to the skillet and cook for 2 minutes until sauce thickens. Pour over the chops and serve.

Calories	Fat	Carbohydrates	Protein	Sodium
277	9g	22g	26g	288mg

Sassy Pork Chops: Quick and Easy, Delectable and Yummy

Serves: 2

Ingredients:

- Ground black pepper [1/4 tsp]
- Reduced-sodium chicken broth [1/4 cup]
- Dried oregano, crushed [1/2 tsp]
- Orange juice [1/4 cup]
- Cooking oil [2 tbsp]
- Chopped onion [1/2 cup]
- Eight pork loin chops (with bone), cut 3/4 inch thick
- Medium red, green, and sweet yellow peppers cut into strips [2 pcs]
- Garlic salt [1/2 tsp]
- Thinly sliced celery [1 cup]

- Chopped chipotle chili peppers in adobo
  sauce [1 tbsp]

Directions:

In a slow cooker, add the celery, onion, and sweet peppers. Set aside. Season the chops with salt and pepper. Place in the skillet and cook over medium heat until brown on both sides. Add the chops to the cooker. Add broth, chipotle peppers, orange juice, and oregano in a bowl. Mix and pour on the chops. Cover the cooker and place the low heat. Cook for 7 hours. Place the chops and veggies on a platter and discard the liquid before serving.

Calories	Fat	Carbohydrates	Protein	Sodium
215	7g	4g	33g	363mg

7 - BEEF RECIPES IDEAL FOR LUNCH AND DINNER

BEEF AND BROCCOLI: A CLASSIC ALL-HIT DISH

Serves: 2

Ingredients:

- Hoisin sauce [3 tbsp]
- Cornstarch [3 tsp]
- Reduced-sodium soy sauce [1 tbsp]
- Garlic, minced [3 cloves]
- Boneless beef top sirloin steak, bias-sliced 1/8-inch thick* [12 oz]
- Reduced-sodium beef broth [3/4 cup]
- Toasted sesame oil [2 tsp]
- Canola oil [1 tbsp]
- Crushed red pepper [1/4 tsp]
- Water [2 tbsp]

- Quartered and halved cherry tomatoes [1 cup]
- Chinese egg noodles or whole wheat vermicelli [4 oz]
- Fresh broccoli [1 lb]

Directions:

Add 2 tsp. Cornstarch, garlic, red pepper, and soy sauce in a bowl and mix. Add the beef and coat with the mixture. Set aside and marinate for 20 minutes. Cook the noodles based on the instructions in the package and do not add salt. Set aside when done. Cut the broccoli into 2 inches, peel and set apart. Prepare the sauce by adding water, hoisin sauce, sesame oil and one tsp cornstarch. Set aside. Heat the oil over medium-high heat in a skillet. Add the beef mixture and stir-fry for 2 minutes until you see the center become less pink. Remove from heat and set aside. Add the beef broth to the skillet and then the broccoli. Let it boil and reduce the heat to medium. Cover the skillet and cook until the broccoli is tender. Add the sauce to the broccoli, cook and stir until it thickens. Add the beef and tomatoes, heat them for a while and serve over the noodles.

Calories	Fat	Carbohydrates	Protein	Sodium
379	14g	39g	26g	532mg

GREEK FETA BURGERS: WHO SAYS YOU CAN'T INDULGE IN BURGERS?

Serves: 1

Ingredients:

- Ground black pepper [1/4 tsp]

- Snipped fresh flat-leaf parsley [1 1/2 tsp]

- Fresh spinach leaves [1/2 cup]

- Crumbled reduced-fat feta cheese [1 tbsp]

- Garlic, minced [1 clove]

- One whole wheat hamburger bun, split and toasted

- Cucumber Sauce

- 90 percent or higher lean ground beef [8 oz]

- Tomato slices [2 pcs]

- Thin slivers red onion

- Ground black pepper [1/8 tsp]

Directions:

Prepare the cucumber sauce and set aside. Combine the cheese, garlic, parsley, ground beef, and pepper in a bowl. Mix and shape into 2-inch thick patties. Cook the patties in a skillet over medium-high heat for about 10 minutes and turn to cook the other side evenly. Line the bun halves with spinach and top it with tomato slices, patties, and sauce. Garnish with red onion and serve.

Calories	Fat	Carbohydrates	Protein	Sodium
292	14g	14g	27g	356mg

GRILLED FLANK STEAK SALAD: ONE RECIPE YOU'D BE GLAD ABOUT

Serves: 1

Ingredients:

- Cherry tomatoes halved [4 pcs]
- Small yellow and red sweet peppers, stemmed, seeded, and halved [2 pcs]
- Small avocado, halved, seeded, peeled, and thinly sliced [1/4]
- Green onions trimmed [2 pcs]
- Cilantro Dressing
- Torn romaine lettuce [2 cups]
- Fresh cilantro sprigs
- Fresh corn, husked and silks removed [1 ear]
- Beef flank steak [8 oz]

Directions:

Divide the dressing into 2 portions then remove the fat from the steak. Score both sides of the steak in a diamond pattern by cutting shallow diagonals at 1-inch distances. Place the steak in a resealable plastic bag and pour the other half of the cilantro dressing. Seal the bag and set aside the remaining dressing. Turn the bag to coat the steak and marinate for 30 mins in the fridge. Coat the corn, sweet pepper, and green onions with cooking spray. Grill the steak and corn on the griller until the steak is cooked as desired and the corn is tender. Turn the steak once to cook both sides evenly. Reduce the heat to medium and add the meat, followed by the veggies after a couple of minutes, on the griller. Cover and then grill. Slice the meat against the grain and chop the sweet peppers and onions. Cut the corn from the cob and leave the kernels in sheets. Serve the meat, veggies, and tomatoes over the lettuce. Drizzle it with the remaining dressing and garnish with cilantro sprigs.

Calories	Fat	Carbohydrates	Protein	Sodium
357	15g	31g	29g	376mg

SUPER LOADED NACHOS: TOP-NOTCH DISH PERFECT FOR SHARING

Serves: 1

Ingredients:

- Homemade Taco Seasoning

- Ground turmeric [1/4 tsp]

- Shredded reduced-fat cheddar cheese [1/2 cup]

- Paprika [1/4 tsp]

- All-purpose flour [1 tbsp]

- Extra-lean ground beef [8 oz]

- Shredded part-skim mozzarella cheese [1/2 cup]

- Eight 6-inch corn tortillas

- Fat-free cream cheese, softened [1 oz]

- Fat-free milk [3/4 cup]

- Unsalted butter [2 tsp]

- Water [1/4 cup]

- Sliced green onions [1/4 cup]

- Chopped tomato [1 cup]

- Fresh jalapeno chile pepper, stemmed, seeded, and thinly sliced [1 pc]

- Snipped fresh cilantro [2 tbsp]

- Chopped green or red sweet pepper [1/2 cup]

- Chunky mild salsa [1/2 cup]

Directions:

Heat the oven to 375 deg. F and line the baking sheet with parchment paper. Cut the tortilla into eight wedges and place it in a single layer on the baking sheet. Coat the wedges with cooking spray and bake until wedges become crisp and golden brown. Set aside. To make the cheese sauce, melt the butter in a saucepan over medium heat. Add the flour and mix well. Add the milk and whisk until smooth. Cook and stir until thick and bubbly. Cook for 2 more minutes and add the cream cheese, paprika, cheddar cheese, mozzarella cheese, and turmeric. Cook over medium heat and stir until cheese is melted and smooth. Reduce heat to low and keep the cheese sauce heated over low heat. Don't forget to stir it. Coat the skillet with cooking spray and place over medium heat. Add the meat and cook until brown. Drain the fat and add in the taco seasoning. Cook for 5 minutes and stir until the water has evaporated. Arrange the tortilla on a serving plate, top with meat, cheese sauce, and the veggies. Serve.

Calories	Fat	Carbohydrates	Protein	Sodium
291	11g	23g	24g	356mg

MEATBALL LASAGNA: GO CRAZY WITH BEEF AND PASTA

Serves: 1

Ingredients:

- Lean ground beef [1 lb]

- Medium green sweet peppers stemmed, seeded and quartered [2 pcs]

- Shredded fresh basil or small fresh basil or oregano leaves

- Dried regular or whole-wheat lasagna noodles

- Snipped fresh flat-leaf parsley [2 tbsp]

- Salt [¼ tsp]

- Lasagna

- Soft whole-wheat breadcrumbs [¾ cup]

- Light ricotta cheese [¾ cup]

- Tomato sauce [3 tbsp]

- Shredded reduced-fat mozzarella cheese, divided [1½ cups]
- Ground black pepper [⅛ tsp]
- Chopped drained roasted red peppers [½ cup]
- Snipped fresh basil [¼ cup]
- Egg, lightly beaten [1 pc]
- Light or low-fat tomato-basil pasta sauce [1½ cups]
- Soft goat cheese (chèvre) or finely shredded Parmesan cheese [¼ cup]

Directions:

Preheat the oven to 350 deg. F and line the pan with foil. Add breadcrumbs, red peppers, egg, basil, parsley, tomato sauce, salt and pepper in a bowl. Add the ground beef and mix. Shape into 24 meatballs and place in a pan. Bake for 20 mins. Prepare the lasagna by increasing the oven temperature to 425 deg F. Line the sheet with foil and place the pepper quarters with the cut-sides down on the sheet. Roast for 20 minutes and do not cover. Wrap it in foil and let it cool for 20 mins. Peel the pepper quarters' skins and set aside. Reduce the oven temperature to 375 deg F. Cook the lasagna noodles based on packaging instructions and drain. Rinse with cold water and remove again then set aside. Add mozzarella, goat, and ricotta cheese in a bowl and mix. Spread half a cup of the pasta sauce on the baking dish. Layer two fo the cooked noodles on the plate. Add the meatballs on top and two more of cooked noodles. Top it with ricotta mixture. Add the peppers and the remaining cooked noodles. Spread the remaining sauce over it. Bake for 50 mins., without cover. Uncover and sprinkle with remaining mozzarella. Baked unclever again for up to ten mins. Let it cool and serve.

Calories	Fat	Carbohydrates	Protein	Sodium
263	8g	22g	23g	468mg

Serves: 4-5

Ingredients:

Beef

- Garlic, minced [2 cloves]

- Lemon juice [1 tbsp]

- Finely shredded lemon peel [1 Tsp

- Olive oil [1 tbsp]

- Ground black pepper [1/4 Tsp

- Snipped fresh oregano [1 tbsp

- Ground cumin [1/2 tsp]

- Salt [1/2 tsp]

- Lean boneless beef top sirloin steak or top loin steak [1 lb]

Sauce

- Fresh oregano leaves [2 tbsp]

- Small shallots, peeled [2 pcs]

- Lemon juice [1 tbsp]

- Packed fresh Italian parsley leaves [1 1/3 cups]

- Olive oil [2 tbsp

- Salt [1/4 tsp]

- Crushed red pepper [1/8 tsp]

- Cider vinegar [2 tbsp]

- Garlic peeled [3 cloves]

Veggies

- Small boiling onions, peeled [8 oz]

- Medium green sweet pepper, cut into 1-1/2 inch pieces [1 pc]

- Whole button mushrooms [8 oz]

Directions:

Remove the fat from the meat and cut it into 1-inch size pieces. Place the meat in a plastic bag and set aside. Add lemon peel, olive oil, lemon juice, cumin, oregano, garlic, salt and pepper in a bowl and mix. Pour them over the meat and seal the bag. Marinate for 24 hours and turn the bag occasionally. Add oil, oregano, parsley, shallots, vinegar, garlic, salt, red pepper, and lemon juice in a blender and blend well. Cover and chill. Cook the onions in a saucepan with boiling water for three mins without lid. Drain and remove the meat from the marinade. Skewer the veggies and meat alternately and brush them with the marinade.

Place the kebabs on the grill, cover and cook for up to 12 minutes and making sure to turn them while grilling. Serve with sauce.

Calories	Fat	Carbohydrates	Protein	Sodium
281	16g	14g	23g	506mg

BEEF AND VEGGIE RAGOUT: A MUST-TRY FRENCH CLASSIC DISH

Serves: 3-4

Ingredients:

- 14 oz can lower-sodium beef broth [2 pcs]
- Cherry tomatoes halved [2 cups]
- Minced garlic [4 cloves)
- Sliced fresh cremini or button mushrooms [3 cups
- Boneless beef chuck roast [1 ½ lbs]
- Port wine or dry sherry [1/2 cup
- Chopped onion [1 cup]
- Salt [1/2 Tsp
- Hot cooked noodles [4 cups]
- Ground black pepper [1/2 tsp]
- Quick-cooking tapioca crushed [1/4 cup]
- Sugar snap peas [4 cups]

Directions

Remove the fat from the meat and cut it into ¾-inch pieces. Lightly coat the skillet with cooking spray and place over medium-high heat. Add the meat and cook until meat is brown. Drain the fat off and set aside. Add the onion, salt, garlic, pepper, and mushrooms in the slow cooker. Sprinkle the tapioca and add the meat. Add the broth or the wine. Cover and cook on low heat for 8 to 10 hours. Add the sugar snap peas. Cover and let it cook for 5 minutes and add the cherry tomatoes. Serve over hot noodles.

Calories	Fat	Carbohydrates	Protein	Sodium
208	4g	19g	24g	401mg

Conclusion

Diabetes type 2, a disease that is known to have killed millions, is not as invincible as it may seem. I understand it takes more than just your physical health to suffer as soon as you get diagnosed. Some people may even suffer emotionally and psychologically as well. However, despite all the medications ready for you to take, all the recipes written in any book, and all the doctors and loved ones willing to help you through the way, nothing is possible unless you pick up the pieces and convince yourself that it is a fight you must face.

It all starts with you, your willingness and your commitment even after everything is said and done. Reversing diabetes takes patience and discipline. Condition yourself to that and be ready for a harsh ride. It's worth fighting for, I assure you.

After this book, you may feel like you need to find out more about your condition so feel free to observe yourself, ask professionals if needed, read books, and do not forget to record your progress and findings.

As for your food, don't let *what you put in your food* hinder you from enjoying it. Just because you have diabetes does not mean you are in for a life without sweetness. Explore the possibilities, and it will surely help you cope and eventually successfully reverse it. Thank you for purchasing this book!

FINAL WORDS

Thank you again for purchasing this book!

I really hope this book is able to help you.

The next step is for you to **join our email newsletter** to receive updates on any upcoming new book releases or promotions. You can sign-up for free and as a bonus, you will also receive our "*7 Fitness Mistakes You Don't Know You're Making*" book! This bonus book breaks down many of the most common fitness mistakes and will demystify many of the complexities and science of getting into shape. Having all this fitness knowledge and science organized into an actionable step-by-step book will help you get started in the right direction in your fitness journey! To join our free email newsletter and grab your free book, please visit the link and signup: **www.hmwpublishing.com/gift**

Finally, if you enjoyed this book, then I would like to ask you for a favor, would you be kind enough to leave a review for this book? It would be greatly appreciated!

Thank you and good luck in your journey!

Sugar Detox

The Ultimate Beginner's Diet Guide Recipes Solution To Sugar Detox Your Body & Quickly Beat the Sugar Cravings Addiction Naturally

By *Simone Jacobs*

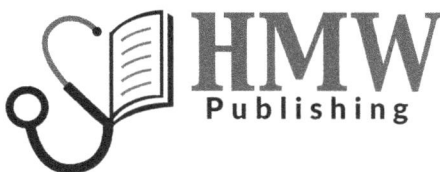

HMW Publishing

For more great books visit:

HMWPublishing.com

Table of Contents

INTRODUCTION

This book contains proven steps and strategies on how you can successfully overcome your sugar addiction. This Sugar Detox guide will help you discover how you can still eat delicious meals and become healthier.

Moreover, you'll learn the advantages of kicking junk, sugary and processed foods out of your life. Likewise, will also explain and reveal how to deal with the symptoms of sugar detox. Lastly, this book will also provide you with delicious meal plans, action plan, and Sugar Detox-friendly recipes to help you get started right away!

Also, before you get started, I recommend you joining our email newsletter to receive updates on any upcoming new book releases or promotions. You can sign-up for free, and as a bonus, you will receive a free gift. Our "*Health & Fitness Mistakes You Don't Know You're Making*" book! This book has been written to demystify, expose the top do's and don'ts and to finally equip you with the information you need to get in the best shape of your life. Due to the overwhelming amount of misinformation and lies told by magazines and self-proclaimed "gurus", it's becoming harder and harder to get reliable information to get in shape. As opposed to having to go through dozens of biased, unreliable and un-trustworthy sources to get your health & fitness information. Everything you need to help you has been broken down in this book for you to easily follow and to immediately get results to achieve your desired fitness goals in the shortest amount of time.

Once again, to join our free email newsletter and to receive a free copy of this valuable book, please visit the link and signup now: www.hmwpublishing.com/gift

CHAPTER 1: SUGAR – THE ROOT OF ALL HEALTH EVIL

Oh, sugar! How do I love thee? Let me count the ways. Studies reveal that the average American consumes about 22.7 teaspoons of sugar daily. Even without adding sugar to your food, you are eating processed foods that are packed with sugar to enhance the flavor and texture of the food and to act as a preservative to extend its shelf life.

To give you a picture, here are the most common food you consume every day and their sugar content:

Food	Size	Amount of sugar (1 teaspoon = 4.2 grams)
Ketchup	3 tablespoons	1.77 teaspoons
Oreo cookies	3 cookies	2.49 teaspoons

Low-fat fruit yogurt	8 ounces	6.16 teaspoons
Cola	1 2 ounces	7.93 teaspoons
Lucky charms	1 cup	2.55 teaspoons
Wheat bread	2 slices	0.66 teaspoons
Pork and beef bologna	4 slices	1.18 teaspoons

The natural foods you eat also contain natural sugar. For example, 27 grams of corn, 1, 135 cups of rice, 454 eggs, and 7 red apples contain 22.7 teaspoons of sugar.

If you are not mindful of what you eat, you can easily consume excessive amounts of sugar than what your body needs. **According to the American Heart Association (AHA), men need 9 teaspoons or 37.5 grams of sugar and women need 6 teaspoons or 25 grams of sugar daily.**

Our bodies need sugar or glucose to function. To

understand the importance of sugar, let's take a quick look at what sugar is and in what forms we need to make it for the best benefits, specifically glucose and fructose.

WHAT IS SUGAR?

Sugar is a pure form of carbohydrate that comes in many ways.

THE SIX (6) KINDS OF SUGAR

* Glucose – occurs naturally in plant juices and fruits. This pure sugar can be carried in the blood. It is the other half of the sucrose or table sugar, paired with fructose.

* Fructose - occurs naturally in cane sugar, fruits, honey, and root vegetables. It is the other half of sucrose, paired with glucose.

* Galactose – combines with glucose to form lactose. This is also known as milk sugar, and it makes up 5 percent of cow's milk.

* Sucrose – or commonly known as table sugar. This sugar naturally occurs in sugar

cane and beets.

- Maltose - made up of two joined glucose molecules.

- High fructose corn syrup – this sugar is chemically very similar to sucrose. However, half of the glucose is converted to fructose.

All carbohydrates, once consumed, are converted into glucose during digestion, which is the sugar that our body needs.

The problem is we consume food with too added sugar. We add table sugar in almost every food we eat – from coffee, tea, baked goods, and more. Table sugar is composed of 50 percent glucose and 50 percent fructose.

Glucose, as mentioned before, is metabolized throughout the body – the glucose is absorbed from the intestines into the bloodstream and then distributed to all the cells of the body. Glucose is vital to the proper functioning of the brain since it is the primary source of fuel of the billions of neural nerve cells in the brain. Neurons can't store glucose themselves, so they need a constant supply from the bloodstream.

BLAME IT ON FRUCTOSE

Fructose is processed mainly by the liver and is turned into fat, which can build up and enter the bloodstream. Moreover, the market is also flooded with products – from soda to soup, with high fructose corn syrup. High fructose corn syrup is cheaper and sweeter than sucrose made from sugar cane and beets. What's the difference? Not enough to fuss about since they both contain fructose and everyone can benefit from eating less, if not eliminating it, from their diet.

When you consume too much fructose, it causes various health risks, including type 2 diabetes, insulin resistance, hypertension, and obesity. In fact, nephrologist Richard Johnson from the University of Colorado Denver, states that when you trace the path of the illness back to its primary cause, you will find your way again to sugar, fructose in particular.

SUGAR ADDICTION: A NOT SO SWEET LOVE STORY

If an extra slice of cake or chocolate has tempted you, then you know exactly how addictive sweets are and how difficult it is to cut back. To put it just, sugar in our bloodstream stimulates the same pleasure centers in the brain that responds to cocaine and heroin.

Sugar is not all bad for us. In fact, our body needs sugar. Johnson theorized that our ancestors evolved to become an efficient processor of fructose for survival, storing even the smallest amounts it as fat during times when food is abundant for use during the scarce seasons. Thus, today, we have a craving for fruit sugar.

For some people, sugar can end up in a full-blown

addiction, the same way someone is addicted to abuse drugs like cannabis, amphetamine, and nicotine. There is no difference. The only dissimilarity is that sugar is legal and is not a controlled substance. In fact, people who are addicted to alcohol and drugs claim that craving for junk and sweet foods is similar. The worst part, sugar is not a regulated product. Often, we consume sugary foods without knowing the risks that it poses to our health.

HOW DOES SUGAR DESTROY US? LET US COUNT THE WAYS.

Sugar is a bad habit, and it's a bad habit that's hard to break. Most of the time, we don't realize that overeating sweets and junk food are not a problem. To give you an idea just how bad sugar is for your health, here are some of their long-term effects.

BAD FOR YOUR TEETH

Added sugar, high fructose corn syrup, and sucrose

contain calories without any essential nutrients. Hence, they are called empty calories – they contain no essential fats, vitamins, minerals, or protein – just pure energy.

When you get 10 to 20 percent or more of your calories from sugar, this can cause nutrient deficiency and health problems.

Sugar is also bad for the teeth because it is a source of digestible energy for the harmful bacteria in the mouth.

CAUSE LIVER PROBLEMS

As mentioned earlier, sugar is broken down into two simple sugars, fructose, and glucose. We need glucose in our body while there is no physiological need for fructose. Moreover, fructose can only be metabolized in the liver, where it is transformed into glycogen and stored in the liver when not used.

It is not a problem if you only eat small amounts of fructose from fruits and you are physically active. However, if you overeat fructose-rich food, you will overload your liver, forcing it to turn the fructose into fat. When you repeatedly eat a significant amount of sugar, it can lead to a non-alcoholic fatty liver and cause various health problems.

Keep in mind that it is almost impossible to overeat fructose from eating fruits since they contain very little fructose. The problem starts when you consume foods with too much sugar additives.

CAUSE INSULIN RESISTANCE AND DIABETES

Insulin is a hormone that is vital to various bodily functions. It helps blood sugar or glucose to enter the cells from the bloodstream. It also tells the cells when to begin burning glucose instead of fat.

When you have high levels of glucose, the body works overtime to produce insulin, flooding the cells with the hormone. Thus, the cells become resistant to it. When you are insulin resistant, it leads to various diseases, including obesity, metabolic syndrome, cardiovascular disease, and especially type II diabetes.

Cause Cancer

Insulin does not only regulate the glucose levels in the body. It also controls the growth and multiplication of cells, which is the characteristic of cancer.

Many scientists believe that if you consume too much sugar, the constant high levels of insulin in the body can cause cancer.

Excessive Weight Gain and Obesity

Not only is fructose metabolized differently from glucose. Studies also show that fructose does not have the same satiety as glucose. People who drank fructose-sweetened beverage felt hungrier and less satiated than people who drank glucose-sweetened drink. Furthermore, the fructose does not lower ghrelin, a hunger hormone, as efficiently as glucose can.

Over time, because fructose isn't as filling, you will feel the need to increase your caloric intake, eating more food, which, in turn, causes weight gain.

Many studies reveal that sugar is the main cause childhood obesity. Kids who drink sugar-sweetened beverages are 60 percent more at risk of obesity. If you want to lose weight, the most important thing you can do is to reduce sugar consumption.

RAISES CHOLESTEROL LEVEL

For a long time, people blamed saturated fat for heart disease, which is the number one cause of death in the world. Recent studies reveal that saturated fat is not to blame. Evidence suggests that SUGAR and not fat, is the leading cause of heart disease, due to the harmful effects of metabolizing fructose.

Studies reveal that high amounts of fructose raise the triglycerides, dense, small low-density lipoprotein and oxidized LDL, increase the levels of glucose in the blood, insulin levels, and abdominal obesity in as short as 10 weeks.

Consequently, various observational studies reveal

a healthy relationship between high sugar consumption and the risk of heart disease.

Aside from the chronic diseases, most of the people who are addicted to sugar experience the following symptoms:

- Heart rate changes

- Mood changes

- Vision changes

- Seizures and convulsions

- Diarrhea

- Poor equilibrium/dizziness

- Weakness and fatigue

- Rash/hives

- Joint pain

- Memory loss

- Headaches and migraines

- Vomiting and nausea

- Insomnia/sleep problems

- Weight-loss problems

With all the health problems that can be traced back to our love for sweet foods, there is a need to detoxify from sugar. Our bodies have evolved to get by with just the smallest amount of fructose. The problem is that our world is flooded with high fructose corn syrup and sucrose. It can be challenging to break up with sugar, but it is an effort that we need to do for our overall health.

Chapter 2: Why You Need to End Your Love Affair with Sugar

Now that you understand how too much sugar and sugar addiction can be detrimental to your health, it is time for detoxification and rehabilitation. It will take considerable effort and willpower to reset your body from a state of chaos. However, rebooting your system will benefit you in the long run.

The Benefits of Sugar Detoxification

Regulate Insulin Production

Mentioned earlier, too much sugar increases the production of insulin, which can often cause insulin resistance and lead to diabetes. Too much fructose also turns into stored fat. When you detoxify, the output of insulin in your body normalizes, which reduces the storage of fat in the belly and food cravings.

IMPROVE THE INSULIN SENSITIVITY

When the body has high levels of insulin all the time, the cells become resistant to it. Thus, the body is unable to regulate blood sugar levels efficiently. Rebooting your system allows the body to adjust the production of insulin, which improves blood sugar regulation, helping you lose weight and improve your health.

NORMALIZES CORTISOL PRODUCTION

Cortisol is a hormone produced by the adrenal glands and the levels of the cortisol in the body rise and fall during different times during the whole day. It is at its highest level in the morning to help you get ready and move at the start the day, and it is at its lowest at night to help you wind down for a good night's rest. When your body has too much blood sugar, it weakens the adrenal glands, which affects cortisol production, a hormone that also helps regulate the blood sugar on a metabolic level.

When the adrenal glands are tired, it is unable to produce the right amount of cortisol that you need in a day. Hence, you will feel sluggish and low in energy. Instinctively, you will want to reach for a quick fix and most of the time. You will munch on a carbohydrate snack, coke, sugary food, or coffee. This is only a temporary solution, one that leads to a spike in blood sugar and insulin production, which later ends up with your blood sugar crashing and ultimately, weakening your adrenal glands even more. The result is a continuous low cortisol production, which is evident in the morning when you wake up feeling tired and unrested even after a night's sleep.

When you detoxify, the system resets, helping your adrenal glands recover and enable it to supply your body with the right amounts of cortisol at different times of the day.

LOWERS THE PRODUCTION OF

GHRELIN, THE HUNGER HORMONE

When you consume sugary food, your body increases its production of insulin so that the sugar can be converted and used by the cells of your body. It also increases the levels of leptin, a hormone that regulates fat storage and appetite, which decreases the production of ghrelin, controlling your food intake. The idea is that when you eat, your body automatically works to let you know that you should feel less hungry.

The problem occurs when you consume too much fructose. The cycle that should tell you that you are full does not happen. You already know that the body uses glucose. Glucose also suppresses the production of ghrelin and stimulates the production of leptin, which both works to suppress the appetite.

Fructose, on the other hand, not only affects the regulation of ghrelin, but it also interferes with the brain's communication with leptin, which leads to overeating. This is why fructose leads to excessive weight gain, insulin resistance, metabolic syndrome, and increased belly fat, as well as the long list of chronic diseases.

When you limit your fructose to healthy levels, it regulates and lowers the production of the hunger hormone ghrelin.

CURES AND PREVENT LEPTIN RESISTANCE

Research reveals that when you consume fructose, you generate more fat in your liver compared to other types of sugar. Moreover, fructose blocks the body's ability to burn fat.

When you eat fewer calories, but you eat large amounts of fructose or your diet is high in sugar it will still cause a fatty liver, insulin resistance, and leptin resistance.

You have learned earlier that when you eat sugar the leptin levels of rising and signal your body that it is full so that you will stop eating. However, when you are leptin resistant, your body no longer responds to leptin. You end up eating more because you don't feel full or satiated. Hence, sugar detoxification will significantly benefit you.

IMPROVES THE EFFECTS OF PEPTIDE YY OR PPY

Peptide YY is a hormone released in the intestines and colon that controls appetite. When the sugar level in your body is unstable of high, it impairs the effects of PYY in appetite suppression.

NATURALLY INCREASES THE LEVELS OF DOPAMINE

Sugary and junk food changes the brain's chemistry, making you want more and more of them, even when you are full. Dr. Robert H. Lustig, pediatric endocrinologist, and Dr. Elissa S. Epel, a psychologist, explain that when you consume large amounts of sugar, your brain releases massive amounts of dopamine, the hormone responsible for making you feel good. When there is a surge of dopamine, it causes the dopamine receptors to down-regulate.Meaning, there are now fewer receptors for them, so the next time you eat sugary and junk foods, their "feel-good" effect is blunted, thus, you need to eat more of them to get the same feeling of reward.

Sugar detoxification resets the reward pathways of the brain, allowing you to feel pleasure from eating real food.

RESETS TASTES BUDS

According to research at the Monell Chemical Senses Center, which was published in the American Journal of Clinical Nutrition, avoiding or eliminating sugar for a period will reboot your taste buds. When you consume low amounts of sugar for a couple of months, even foods with little sugar will taste sweet. This means that when you detoxify, you will be able to enjoy delicious treats more, you will be quickly satisfied with a smaller amount, and you will be less likely to overeat.

REDUCE INFLAMMATION

If you can recall your biology lesson about inflammation, you will remember that our bodies depend on temporary swelling to help fight infections and injuries – the inflammation cleans cellular debris, kill pathogens, and create protection to help to heal. Inflammation of a wound is a symptom that indicates the body has it is doing its job, the swelling, redness, slight tenderness, and warm feeling is the body's defense at work.

However, when the inflammatory response is turned on all the time? When you experience chronic inflammation, the immune system attacks normal cells by mistake, and the process that normally helps the body heals causes destruction.

Dave Grotto, RD, a spokesperson for the American Dietetic Association says the sugar cause inflammatory disease. When the body is unable to regulate the sugar and insulin levels in the body, a hidden inflammation in the body can cause chronic infections. When the blood sugar is high, the body generates more free radicals that damage the cells of the body, stimulating a response from the immune system, which causes inflammation that you cannot see.

Eliminating sugar, processed foods, and ordinary food sensitives, together with consuming foods that help fight off inflammation, reduce your risk of developing chronic diseases.

BOOSTS DETOXIFICATION

As mentioned in the previous benefit, too much sugar in the body increases free radicals. When you detoxify, you not only reduce the damage to your cells caused by free radicals, you also help your body get rid of other toxins that make you fat.

The benefits you get from detoxifying from sugar, as well as processed food, will help your body heal. When you avoid sugar, you will not only lose weight, but you will also benefit from the long-term health improvements.

Food You Need to Avoid

That is the question. To get the full benefit of sugar detoxification, you will not only need to avoid sugar. You will also need to avoid other types of food.

Sugar

By this point, you probably know why you need to cut back on sugar. However, it can be a scary change, especially if you have a sweet tooth. Don't worry; you won't go crazy during your detoxification. Even the most stubborn cravings and addictions will be curved. People who already detoxed claim the incredible change in as little as 24 hours and their desires have lessened

Grains and Gluten

Gluten is the two most common food sensitivities. Most people do not realize that they are sensitive to certain foods because this condition is not a real allergy like shellfish or peanut allergy, which creates hives, close the throat, swell the tongues, and can kill the person within minutes.

Unlike true allergies, food sensitivity is a subtle reaction to food. It is hidden because the small changes usually occur in the digestive tract. When you have food sensitivities, the lining in the gastrointestinal tract, particularly the intestine gradually becomes damaged and porous, a condition called a leaky gut, wherein food particles enter the bloodstream, creating a response to the body's immune system.

Earlier, I have mentioned about how the body protects itself and inflammation is a good sign that the body's defenses are working. However, when you have a leaky gut, your body is consistently in a state of low-grade inflammation as a reaction to the foreign particles in your bloodstream, resulting in many various symptoms that you would not connect to the food you eat. Some of these symptoms include brain fog, fatigue, depression, headaches, sinus problems, allergies, reflux, irritable bowel, autoimmune disease, joint pain, and skin diseases, such as eczema and acne.

Moreover, low-grade inflammation also triggers

insulin resistance, which causes weight gain.

Gluten, a protein found in oats, spelled, rye, barley, and wheat. Some people are unable to digest it, causing a leaky gut. Additionally, because of genetic modification, a new strain of wheat has been created. This grain contains amylopectin A, a super-starch that triggers spikes in blood sugar. Two slices of bread made from this new corn raise the blood sugar more than 2 tablespoons of table sugar.

Gluten sensitivity, together with super-starch, triggers more inflammation, which increases the risk of diabetes and obesity.

All grains, including cereals, bread, and snacks, even the gluten-free kind, can spike blood sugar and insulin because they contain carbohydrates.

Moreover, research shows that when you eat high carb food, mainly if you have been consuming high-fructose food and your liver has been metabolizing fructose for quite some time, even when there is no fructose in your diet, your liver will convert the glucose, found in flour and bread, into fructose. Hence, during your detox, as mentioned earlier, you will need to avoid high carb food, such as rice, bread, and another non-vegetable carbohydrate.

FACTORY-MADE AND PROCESSED FOODS

As you already know, these foods are packed with artificial sweeteners and high-fructose corn syrup. They also made with preservatives, chemicals, additives, monosodium glutamate or MSG, and hydrogenated fats. MSG cause insulin spike, leading to cravings, hunger, and overeating.

During your detox, eat only food that is low-glycemic, contain good fats, proteins, phytonutrients, fiber, minerals, and vitamins.

Keep in mind; MSG can be hidden, so watch out for these ingredients:

- Any "flavoring" or "flavors."

- Anything with "enzyme modified."

- Anything with "hydrolyzed."

- Anything containing "enzymes."

- Anything with "glutamate" in it

- Autolyzed plant protein

- Autolyzed yeast

- Barley malt

- Bouillon and broth

- Carrageenan

- Gelatin

- Glutamate

- Glutamic acid

- Hydrolyzed plant protein (HPP)

- Hydrolyzed vegetable protein (HVP)

- Malt extract

- Maltodextrin

- Natural seasonings

- Protease

- Stock

- Textured protein

- Umami

- Vegetable protein extract

- Yeast extract

- Yeast food or nutrient

- Processed and Refined Vegetable Oils

You will need to avoid sunflower, canola, soybean oil, and more. They contain omega-6 fatty acids that cause inflammation. During your detox, use extra-virgin coconut butter or extra-virgin olive oil. Extra-virgin olive oil contains polyphenols, a potent antioxidant, and anti-inflammatory compounds while coconut butter contains anti-inflammatory fats, such as lauric acid, the same fat found in breast milk. If you need oil for high-heat cooking, grape seed oil is safe.

ALCOHOL

Alcohol is sugar in various forms. Moreover, when you drink alcohol, it impairs self-control, so you will be most likely to overeat mindlessly. It also contains 7 calories per gram, more than the four calories per gram of sugar. It not only causes leaky gut, but it also inflames the liver.

CAFFEINE

Some claim that caffeine speed up metabolism in a process called thermogenesis. However, you will also get the same effect by adding spices to your dishes, such as cayenne or jalapeno pepper. Caffeine is also addictive, and when inserted into sugary drinks, you will crave for more of that food. It also increases hunger. Like sugar, caffeine causes a surge of dopamine and then it wears off eventually. Even if you do not crave for coffee, you will undoubtedly desire for more sugar.

Avoiding caffeine will reboot your system, normalize brain chemistry and lessen cravings. Even decaf contain caffeine, so it is also off limits.

Starting Your Sugar Detoxification:

What Foods to Eat

When you've removed the bad stuff, now is the time to add the proper definite replacement. All the elements of your detox help your body detoxify, shed excess weight, and heal. Avoiding the bad stuff and eating more of the excellent material optimize and accelerate your results.

Detox Pathway Boosters

To maximize your detox, you need to eat more superfoods and foods rich in phytonutrients. When your body is healthy, detoxification is smooth. When your body is toxic, especially when it's flooded with fructose, the liver gets sluggish, detox is slow, and certain toxins remain active longer than the system can handle. Hence, you get sick, and metabolism slows down. It also causes bloating, puffiness, and fluid retention.

When you are overweight, your body is high in

toxins. As you lose weight during sugar detox, the toxins are released out from your fat tissues, and you will need to flush them out. Otherwise, it can impair weight loss and poison your metabolism.

Here are the foods the speed up detox:

1. Watercress

2. Wakame

3. Rosemary

4. Parsley

5. Onion

6. Lemon

7. Kombu

8. Kale

9. Ginger

10. Garlic

11. Eggs

12. Collards

13. Cilantro

14. Cayenne pepper

15. Cauliflower

16. Cabbage

17. Brussels sprouts

18. Broccoli

19. Bok Choy

20. Arame

They are rich in vitamin A and C, B vitamins, antioxidants, and phytonutrients.

Anti-Inflammatory Foods

Inflammation is your body's typical reaction to heal wounds and fight off bacteria. This is what happens when you have a sore throat, a cut, or strain. When the injury is infected, it turns, hot, red, and tender.

The inflammations that you need to be concerned about are the ones hidden inside your body and do not necessarily hurt. It's the inflammation caused by allergens, toxins, stress, bad food, the overgrowth of harmful bacteria in your gut, and low-grade infections.

Anything that causes inflammation will eventually cause insulin resistance, which produces belly fat and your body to hold on to fat cells. Earlier, I have mentioned the food that you need to avoid. Now I am going to give you the list of foods that will help minimize inflammation.

Omega 3 fatty acid-rich foods, such as:

1. Salmon

2. Eggs

3. Grass-fed beef

4. Hemp seeds

5. Chia seeds

6. Walnuts

7. Flaxseeds

8. Spices and herbs, such as turmeric

9. Berries

10. Dark-green leafy vegetables

11. Extra-virgin olive oil

12. Avocado

13. Organic poultry

14. Wild seafood

15. Non-GMO tempeh and tofu

Foods That Cure Leaky Gut and Improve Gut Function

Every individual has 500 species of bacteria in the digestive system. These bacteria help control metabolism, digestion, and inflammation. Research studies also indicate that your weight may be controlled more by that the bacteria in your gut eat than what you eat yourself.

The bacteria in your gut increase, depending on what you eat and feed them. When you eat healthy food, the right bacteria grow and help boost your metabolism. However, if you eat junk, unhealthy diet, the harmful bacteria is the once that increase. This is something you should avoid because bad bacteria produce nasty gas and toxins that cause inflammation, weight gain, puffiness, bloated belly, and diabesity or the metabolic dysfunction. This is characterized by metabolic syndrome, insulin resistance, obesity, and type 2 diabetes, which is all caused by high blood sugar and can be treated using the same treatment.

When there is an imbalance of gut bacteria in your digestive system, it damages the lining of your gut or a leaky gut, which causes inflammation, and in turn, damages metabolism, affects how the brain controls appetite, leads to insulin resistance, and of course, weight gain.

Low sugar, low starch, high fiber, and whole food diet feeds the good bacteria and starves the harmful bacteria. Foods that are rich in minerals and vitamins help improve gut function. It includes:

1. Bok Choy

2. Pumpkin seeds

3. Kale

4. Arugula

5. Carrots

6. Tomatoes

7. Turkey

8. Salmon

9. Chicken

10. Parsley

11. Onion

12. Kimchi

These foods are high in vitamin A, zinc, antioxidants, amino acids, and probiotics.

Blood Sugar Balancers

The key to balance blood sugar is protein. Each meal should contain lean, preferably organic, animal protein, paired with delicious vegetables.

If you are a vegan or a vegetarian, you may have a serious weight and health problem when you substitute meat with starchy food, such as pasta, rice, bread, and other dense carbohydrate food, when once consumed turn into sugar and lead to cravings.

Even beans and grains can be a problem since these foods spike blood sugar and insulin more than animal protein. Eating all veggies can be unhealthy unless you know what you are doing.

Yes, you need to eat less factory-farmed meat, but animal-based protein is important for most people. If they come from pasture-raised or wild sources, then animal protein can be very healthy.

Your detox will partially depend on your current metabolism and health. The sicker you are, the less room you have regarding the sugar you can consume. As you detoxify and lose weight, your resilience will increase, and after the detox period, you can experiment with beans and grains as a source of protein. However, if you currently have significant health concerns, then avoid them, for the time being.

Seeds and nuts are the exceptions when it comes to protein from plant sources. They do not spike blood sugar and are great as snacks if you do not have nut allergies. They are particularly suitable for people with diabesity since they reduce the risk of diabetes, help with weight loss, and improve metabolism since they are packed with good fats, protein, minerals, such as zinc and magnesium, and fiber, all help reverse diabesity.

EXERCISE

Exercise is vital during your detox period. As little as 30 minutes of moderate exercise to begin your day will jump-start your metabolism and balance your hormones, blood sugar, and brain chemistry so that you can make better food choices during the day.

Exercise regulates appetite, reduces cravings, improves insulin sensitivity, and activates detox pathways to help eliminate toxins that cause weight gain, reduce inflammation, reduce stress hormone cortisol, and encourages better help.

Exercise is the best anxiety and depression treatment. It improves self-esteem, well-being, and energy.

If you already have an exercise routine, just continue to do whatever it is you enjoy for 30 minutes. If you haven't been exercising regularly, start with a 30-minute slow or brisk walking. If you can only do 5 minutes, then start with it and do it 2 times a day. Work your way up from there. Walking is the easiest and the most accessible exercise to everyone. It doesn't require any fancy equipment or memberships. You can also try out other physical activities.

SUPPLEMENTS

When it comes to health and weight loss, nutrients are vital. When the body is low in essential nutrients, it craves more food, seeking to get the nutrients it needs. Hence, you end up eating more, often sugary and junk foods, searching for the nutrients that are just not there. You overeat, but the body is still starving and not satisfied.

When you start to eat more real food, you will feel more satisfied, and you will eat less. However, your body will still need the essential amount of high-quality nutrients to help your body efficiently work. Sufficient amount of vitamins and minerals are required to burn calories, regulate appetite, boost detoxification, lower inflammation, regulate cortisol or stress hormones, aid digestion, and help the cells become more sensitive to insulin.

HYDRATE

Most of us are frequently dehydrated. We become even more dehydrated because most of us love to drink caffeinated drinks. Staying hydrated is one of the keys to detoxification. Fluid helps flush out environmental and metabolic toxins through the kidneys, increases energy, and improves regular bowel movements. Thus, drinking at least 8 glasses of water daily is essential during and after detox.

Studies reveal that we often mistake thirst for hunger, and eat instead of drinking. Always keep a bottle of fresh filtered water throughout the day and drink. Hydrate!

WRITE YOUR EXPERIENCE

Keeping a journal and writing down your thoughts, feelings, and experiences unfiltered have been proven to reduce stress and help the process of detoxification. It's one of the best ways to stop the cycle of mindless eating. Journaling enables you to process your emotions and thoughts in a healthy, proactive way rather than just stuffing them down with bad habits and bad foods.

Writing will help you metabolize not just your thoughts, but also your calories better. Keeping an honest account of your experience is essential. Buy a blank notebook and write about your experience every morning and at night.

UNWIND AND RELAX

Most of us are not motivated to take a break seriously. Consider this then: when the body is stressed, it causes a spike in insulin level, increase the level of cytokines or the immune system messenger molecules that cause inflammation, and increase the level of cortisol that causes accumulation of fat on the belly.

Stress also makes you hungrier and increases your cravings for sugar and carbohydrates, which trigger metabolic dysfunction, leading to excessive weight gain. So take time unwind and take a break. The breathing exercise below will help you relax.

5-Minute Relaxation Breathing

1. Sit down as comfortably as you can – on a chair, cross-legged on a cushion on the floor, or on a propped up pillows on your bed.

2. Close your mouth and eyes.

3. Breathe slowly through your nose, counting

to 5 as you inhale.

4. Hold in 5 counts.

5. Slowly exhale, counting to 5 as you breathe out.

6. Repeat for 5 minutes.

GET INTO THE RHYTHM

Whether we like it or not, our bodies evolved into biological organisms. Whether we listen to the signals that our body is sending us or not, it follows a specific rhythm – time to sleep, wake up, eat, relax, and exercise.

Simple behavioral changes will help you get back into the rhythm, which has powerful effects, including better sleep, increased energy, weight loss, and a lot more. Thus, during your detox period, create a schedule and stick to it.

Research shows that eating very late, skipping meals, and not eating breakfast screw up your metabolism. Not eating during the day results in the night-eating syndrome or binge eating at night or getting up in the middle of the night to feed. This causes diabesity, which results in blood sugar swings.

Wake up, sleep, eat, exercise, and relax the same time every day during your detox period. You will soon notice your body getting into the rhythm. The best thing about routines is that you won't have to waste mental energy continually planning your day. Eating an early breakfast will kick-start your metabolism and allow it to burn calories all day. Likewise, you need to avoid eating 2-3 hours before bedtime to prevent fat from being stored while you sleep. While you sleep, your body grows, rebuilds, and repairs itself. However, when you are sleeping, you are burning less energy, so the last thing you want is your belly growing.

GET ENOUGH SLEEP

Not getting sufficient sleep is linked to various diseases, including obesity. Since the invention of the light bulb, humans have been staying up longer and later because we can, which disrupts the body's sync with the natural rhythm of the seasons and mess up with the first sleep pattern.

If you don't get the right amount of sleep, it increases the production of ghrelin, the hunger hormone and it decreases the production of leptin, the appetite-suppressing hormone. When it comes to sugar, sleep is a natural appetite suppressant.

If you are working night shifts, you may have noticed that you are always craving for something sweet, like ice cream, cookies, and more. Your body is not getting enough energy because you are not getting enough sleep, so you eat to get the energy your body needs.

Now that you know what you need to avoid and what you need to get more of; let's get you ready to start your sugar detox.

CHAPTER 3: PREPARING FOR SUGAR DETOX

The key to a successful sugar detoxification is a good plan and efficient preparation. Admit it; you probably spend more time planning vacations and parties than planning how to be healthy. Before you begin your detox, design your life for success and create an environment that will automatically direct you to make healthier choices. For instance, if you have nuts instead of donuts in your pantry, then you are more likely to make a healthy decision. Set your kitchen, your mind, and your school or work environment to maximize your detox. This is Day 1 and Day 2 – the unofficial start of your sugar detox.

SUGAR DETOX YOUR KITCHEN

Your kitchen is probably packed with processed, sugar-packed, and junk food. You are going to start your detox with your kitchen. Throw away any items that fall under the following categories:

1. Packaged, boxed, canned, or anything that is not real food. You can keep anything that is canned whole food, such as artichokes or sardines that contains a couple of real ingredients, such as salt or water.

2. Drinks or foods that contain any form of sugar, including artificial sweeteners, organic cane juice, maple syrup, agave, molasses, and honey, mainly any fruit juices or beverages sweetened with sugar.

3. Foods that contain refined vegetable oils, such as soybean or corn oil, and hydrogenated oil.

4. Foods with dyes, coloring, additives, preservatives, or artificial sweeteners – anything that is processed in any way and has a label.

If you are unsure if the food or drink cuts, the best thing to do is get rid of it. Be thorough!

The following items also need to go. If you don't want to throw them, transfer them somewhere that is far from your eyesight during your detox. You need to avoid them while you are detoxifying. After your detox your body, you may introduce some them back into your diet.

- Products with gluten, including, pasta, bread, bagels, etc.

- All grains, including the ones that are gluten-free.

SUPPLY YOUR KITCHEN WITH THE GOOD STUFF

GROCERIES

After clearing out your cabinets and fridge, it's time to fill them with real, whole, fresh food for your detox.

Make sure you have these staples.

- Almond meal

- Anti-inflammatory and Detoxifying herbs and spices, including turmeric, thyme, cayenne pepper, rosemary, cumin, chili powder, sage, onion powder, oregano, cinnamon, cilantro, coriander, parsley, and paprika

- Apple cider vinegar

- Balsamic vinegar

- Black pepper (peppercorns that you can freshly grind)

- Broth, low-sodium (chicken or vegetable)

- Coconut butter, extra-virgin, also known as coconut oil – it may be solid or liquid at room temperature

- Coconut milk, full-fat, canned

- Dijon mustard

- Jarred or canned Kalamata olives

- Nut butter (raw if possible; choose from almond, cashew, macadamia, or walnut)

- Nuts: almonds, walnuts, macadamia pecans,

- Olive oil, extra-virgin

- Other healthy oils that you like (walnut, sesame, grapeseed, flax, or avocado)

- Sea salt

- Seeds: chia, hemp, pumpkin, flax, sesame

- Tahini or sesame seed paste—great for salad dressings and in sauces for vegetables)

- Tamari, low-sodium, gluten-free

- Unsweetened almond or hemp milk

Depending on the meal plan or the dishes, you plan to prepare for the day or the week during your detox, add the specific ingredients needed; you may not need some of the ingredients listed above. Read on through the recipes, plan your meals, and then shop for the ingredients that you need.

You may think that buying fresh, whole, good food is expensive. However, if you consider how much money you spend on takeout food, convenience food, sodas, coffee, and junk food, you would be surprised that you are spending that much money on food that is toxic. You should also consider how much you would be paying treating diseases brought on by processed and poisonous foods. When you look at the long-term benefits on your health and wallet, choosing healthy foods is way better and healthier for you.

DETOXIFYING BATH SUPPLIES

Relaxing at home is easy. Lavender oil, baking soda, and Epsom salt in your bath soak will not only help you relax; the combination creates a detoxifying and relaxing routine.

For each session, you will need the following:

- 2 cups Epsom salt

- 1/2 cup baking soda

- 10 drops lavender oil

Fill the tub with water as hot as you can handle. Add the Epsom salt, baking soda, and lavender oil. To make the bathroom more relaxing, you can play some soothing music and light candles. Soak in the tub for about 20-30 minutes.

This detoxifying bath will help you de-stress and relax for a better sleep. Your muscles and mind will benefit from this healing bath.

SUGAR DETOX JOURNAL

Purchase a journal or notebook. Here you will record your experiences, thoughts, and results.

SUPPLEMENTS

Most people are deficient in necessary nutrients,

especially people who haven't been taking care of their bodies. Before you start your detox, make sure you have the following on hand. They will supply your body with the essential nutrients that it needs. The combination is designed for long-term usage. You can find any of the supplements at your local health store.

Supplement	Dosage	Benefits
Alpha lipoic acid (ALA)	300-600 milligrams	Balances insulin and blood sugar; taken together with other supplements that optimize metabolism, blood sugar balance, and insulin.

Chromium	500-1000 micrograms	Balances insulin and blood sugar; taken together with other supplements that optimize metabolism, blood sugar balance, and insulin.
Cinnamon	500-1000 milligrams	Balances insulin and blood sugar; taken together with other supplements that optimize metabolism, blood sugar balance, and insulin.
Green tea catechins	100-200 milligrams	Balances insulin and blood sugar; taken together with other supplements that optimize metabolism, blood sugar balance, and insulin.

Magnesium citrate	200-300 milligrams (2 - 3 capsules) 1-2 times a day	This is used to manage constipation caused by PolyGlycopleX or PGX, mainly if your stomach is not used too much fiber. This also helps improve sleep, reduce anxiety, improve the control of blood sugar, and help cure muscle cramps.
Multivitamin and multimineral supplement	Take as indicated on the label	Help run the metabolism, improve insulin functioning, and balance blood sugar.

PolyGly copleX or PGX (capsules or powder)	2.5 - 5 grams before every meal; you can take additional doses during the day to control cravings	This super fiber slows down insulin and blood sugar spikes. It also reduces needs and makes you feel full longer. Take before every meal with a large-sized glass of water. The powder form works better than the capsule. This will also help you manage night eating or night cravings. Drink the recommended eight glasses water daily to ensure the fiber moves through your body.
Purified fish oil (DHA/ EPA)	2 grams	Balances blood sugar, sensitize insulin, anti-inflammatory, boosts brain function and prevents heart disease.

Vitamin D3	2,000 IU	
Zinc	1 5 - 3 0 milligrams	Balances insulin and blood sugar; taken together with other supplements that optimize metabolism, blood sugar balance, and insulin.

TESTING TOOLS TO MONITOR YOUR PROGRESS

If you have the money or if your budget allows, you may want to get the following tools that will help you test and monitor your progress.

- A glucose monitor

- A weighing scale, preferably one who uploads your weight, body composition, and BMI; if possible, one that directly uploads your info to a smartphone.

- A blood pressure monitor, if possible, one that instantly uploads your info into a smartphone

- A personal movement track to track your daily sleep and activity

EXERCISE CLOTHING

The goal here is for maximum success. You will be more likely to exercise if you keep a pair of appropriate exercise clothing and your supplies in the same place. Whenever you are ready to go, you have everything you need. Get your sneakers out of the closet or buy a new pair. Choose to clothe that you are most comfortable with. Remove any obstacles so that when you start your detox, you are ready to go.

WATER FILTER AND BOTTLE

The best way to drink pure, clean water is to filter your own using a simple carbon and then pour the water into a glass or stainless steel bottle. You can find these items in the supermarket or at the home-goods store.

REDUCE CONSUMPTION OF SUGAR, CAFFEINE, AND ALCOHOL

The 2-day preparation is the start of your detox, and during this period, you will start weaning yourself off from the sugar, alcohol, and caffeine. These substances will make you feel temporarily alert and energized, but their effects wear off fast and you'll end up in a vicious crash-and-crave cycle.

- It won't be easy getting off caffeine. Do it in stages. Reduce your usual amount to half during the first day, and then reduce again by half the second day. During the official first day of your detox, go cold turkey. Take a nap if you are tired. Lots of water, a gentle exercise, a hot bath, and 1, 000 mg twice daily of vitamin C can help reduce any a headache that you may experience because of withdrawal.

- Day 2 is the time to quit alcohol and any beverage that is sweetened with artificial sweeteners or sugar. This is also the time to stop eating processed food.

How Do I Deal with Detox Symptoms

During this phase, you have already started weaning yourself from sugar and processed foods so that you may feel hungry. You will also experience the typical signs of hunger, such as a vacant sensation in the chest or abdominal area and belly growling. You will crave for sweets and feel fatigued or light-headed between meals, have trouble completing a 30-minute walk, want for coffee, experience brain fog or have difficulty concentrating, and feel anxious, moody, or short-tempered.

Rest

Relax, nap, and rest. This is vital during the first few days of detox. Rest relaxes your nervous system, the system responsible for your fight or flight response during a stressful event, helps the body repair. The first 2 days of your detox are where detoxification magic happens. Your body will adjust, and you will feel less than great, so you need to rest. This will pass once your body has transitioned.

Accept the Detox Symptoms

Feeling not so great is a great sign. It means that your body is transitioning and eliminating the toxins from your body.

Flush the Toxins

Take a detoxifying bath, get a massage, enjoy a sauna, do stretching or a gentle yoga. All these things will help reduce inflammation and increase circulation in your body, which helps reduce soreness and achiness, increase chemical secretion, move toxins, and purify the body.

Get Things Moving

Clean bowels that efficiently working prevents constipation and headaches. Here are some tips to get things moving

- Drink lots of water to flush the kidneys and clean the intestines.

- Add 2 tablespoons ground flax seeds into your soups, salads, or shakes. These are rich in fiber and absorb plenty of water.

- Take 100-150 mg of magnesium citrate twice daily will help regular bowel movement. You can take as much as 6 capsules. Stop taking or reduce the amount if the bowel becomes too loose.

- Take 1000-2000 mg vitamin C one to two times daily.

- Drink an herbal laxative, such as senna, cascara, or rhubarb before bedtime.

- Exercise helps things get moving. It's a powerful bowel stimulant and

- Sweat it out. Intense activity helps you sweat, which releases toxins through your skin. If your exercise does not cause you to sweat, take an infrared or steam sauna.

- Use an enema or suppository. There are available medications that you can buy at your local drugstore.

- Try liquid magnesium citrate. This is usually used to flush the bowel before a colonoscopy. If you can find this at your local drugstore, then you can use it. However, this solution is compelling. It can make you go in less than 4 hours, so don't leave the house and be ready.

- When all else fail, then it's time to see your doctor and find out what else is going on.

Move Your Body

A gentle exercise will help your circulation moving, flushing toxic fluid. Here's a simple yet effective way that can make a huge difference. Lie on your back close to a wall. Put your legs straight up against the wall and let it stay there for 20 minutes.

Take 2000 mg buffered vitamin C

One to two capsules daily will help relieve the detox symptoms.

Drink Lots of Fluids

Ensure that you are drinking a minimum of 8 glasses every day. You can also drink herbal teas if desired.

Eat!

Eat a lot when you are feeling it. Eat as much of the following non-starchy vegetables:

- Zucchini

- Watercress

- Turnip greens

- Tomatoes

- Swiss chard

- Summer squash

- Spinach

- Snow peas

- Snap beans

- Shallots

- Radishes

- Radicchio

- Parsley

- Palm hearts

- Onions

- Mustard greens

- Mushrooms

- Lettuces

- Kale

- Jalapeño peppers

- Green beans

- Gingerroot

- Garlic

- Fennel

- Endive

- Eggplant

- Dandelion greens

- Collard greens

- Chives

- Celery

- Cauliflower

- Cabbage

- Brussels sprouts

- Broccoli

- Bell peppers (red, green, yellow)

- Beet greens

- Bean sprouts

- Asparagus

- Arugula

- Artichoke

Don't Forget Your Snacks

To keep the hunger and craving away, include 2 snacks in your meal plan. A small protein-based dish with fiber and healthy fats, like sugar-free spreads or dips with veggies or nuts will help keep your energy up and your blood sugar steady. You can also cook your meals, adding a bit of extra to serve as your snack - snack doesn't necessarily mean nuts and spread. If you want, you can eat six small meals a day – some people find this easier.

SET YOUR MIND

You have to set your mind right. If you are thinking wrong and if you feel that you won't succeed, then you will head that way. It's not just healthy eating habits; it's also a positive mindset that will determine the success of your detox.

Your journal will help you root out your beliefs, attitudes, and mental obstacles that are preventing you from success. You need to be aware of the challenges so that you can shift your focus to what you want to achieve and how you can reach it.

During your 2-day preparation, focus on the questions below and write whatever comes to your mind. If other feelings and thoughts go to you when you are writing down your answers, then write them down as well. Writing down what happens to your mind makes you more accountable to yourself, and it can transform your inner desires into reality. Here are the questions that you need to answer.

- Why am I detoxifying? What can I achieve in my life and my body with this detox?

- What three particular goals do I want to achieve during this detox?

- What are three particular things stopping me from achieving my weight goal? Is it sugar addiction? Emotional eating? Busy life? Always eating junk food? Fear of failure? Fear of success? Food pushers who advertise and encourage unhealthy food and eating habits?

- What beliefs hinder me from being healthy? Do I think I don't deserve much attention and time? Do I have this belief that being healthy is hard? I tried before, and it wasn't successful.

- Was it the way I overeat? Was it the way I eat food that is not nourishing?

- How do sickness and excess weight affect my ability to fulfill the things I want to do and make me happy?

- If I start eating healthy, how will my life change? If I take care of my health, how will it affect my life?

- How was my life when I was healthier and nurtured myself with care?

The more the obstacles and the benefits come into life, the better you will be able to get past them.

81

More than that, the more connected you are to your intention and purpose, the more motivated you will be.

Be honest with yourself. Why are you detoxifying? Who are you doing this for? For yourself? For your loved ones? How different will your life be if you are healthy? The most important questions of all – will you be there to witness your children and grandchildren grow up? How long will you be able to spend time with your family and friends?

MEASURE YOUR PROGRESS

The day before you start your detox, measure the following and record them in your detox journal.

WEIGHT

Without clothes on, weigh yourself the very first thing in the morning when you wake up.

HEIGHT

Measure how tall you are in feet and inches.

Waist Size

Wrapping the tape measure around your belly button, measure the widest point of your waist, not the portion where your belt is located.

Hip Size

Same with the waist, measure the widest point around your hips.

Thigh Circumference

Same with the waist and hips, measure the widest point around each, individual thigh.

Blood Pressure

If you have a blood pressure cuff, then you can do this at home. If not, this can be done at the drugstore or by your doctor.

Now you are ready to start your sugar detox.

Chapter 4: What to Expect and How to Get Through

You are officially starting your sugar detoxification – Day 3 to Day 14. It won't be an easy adjustment and transition. However, if you armed with the knowledge of what to expect and how to tips on how you can deal with the various symptoms, your journey will be more comfortable.

Day 3: This Is It!

This is the when most people usually experience flu-like symptoms, self-doubt, and low blood sugar. This is the start a very challenging journey. Hold on to your reigns! You are likely not experiencing real cold or flu, but you are experiencing the symptoms of sugar detox -this is a typical reaction, and it will subside after a couple of days.

Day 4: Ten More Days to Go!

You may notice your skin breaking out with pimples. This is a normal and a great sign! Your detoxification is working, and your body is clearing out the toxins. You may also experience minor irritation on your skin and mood changes.

Day 5: I made it Through!

The cravings and the headaches will start to go away. If you are unprepared for hunger, slip-ups and temptations may happen. This is what your preparation is all about – having the right food and healthy snacks on hand, plus planning meals on time.

Day 6: Almost Half Way Done!

The flu or cold-like symptoms will begin to subside on this day. You can also check out your supply. The meal plans you have created, and the recipes to make sure you are still on point. It's also good to read the preparation tips once more.

DAY 7: ONE WEEK DOWN!

This is where most people experience diarrhea, constipation, or bloating. Make sure you follow the tips given on how to avoid constipation.

DAY 8: ONE MORE WEEK!

Over the weekend, you may feel the temptation and slip-off from your detox. If you haven't experienced fatigue early on, then this may be the day you will start to feel worn-out. You might start feeling tired of the food that you are eating and feel overwhelmed by how much preparation you need to do for your food.

If you slipped, don't be harsh on yourself. Instead, be more firm in your commitment. The recipes included in this book are also easy, and there are too many sugar-detox recipes online. Just make sure each recipe follows the guidelines mentioned above.

Day 9: Yeah! I Am Feeling Good! No More Cravings!

Gas, bloating, and other digestive issues will begin to clear. You may have collected a couple of recipes that you'd like to try and you are getting the hang of cooking. You can change and add any recipes you have clipped outside of this book into your meal plan.

You will also notice that you are no more extended craving more junk and sweet foods the way you did before you started detoxifying. Read your journal. Look back at your successes and your struggles. Your daily log will show you how far you have gone.

Day 10: I Feel A Bit Weak, But This Is Not As Hard As I Thought. I Should Continue Eating Healthy!

A low carb diet can result in weakness or shakiness.

If you have been regularly working out, you will notice your performance is affected. Make sure you are getting enough healthy fat. This will be your primary source of energy since you have cut back on carbohydrates and sugar.

After the feeling of lethargy, you will feel the improvement in your energy and mood as you approach the end of your detox. You've now learned to surf on sugar-free waves.

DAY 11: I SLEEP LIKE A BABY, BUT I AM CRAVING FOR SOMETHING SWEET

By this day, you may notice that you are sleeping faster and better. You will also see that you feel refreshed and rested when you wake up in the morning. Ensure that you follow your waking and sleeping schedule.

However, you may feel the longing for the junk and sugary foods you usually eat, and you may get bored with the food choices. The excitement may pan out at eating healthy food. Again, search for more exciting sugar detox-friendly recipes. You can certainly add tons of recipes to your 2-week meal plan. You can even continue eating healthy for life!

DAY 12: AM I LOSING ANY WEIGHT? THE TWO WEEKS ARE ALMOST UP.

The sugar detox will help you shed the excess weight, but it won't help if you weigh yourself every day. It's ideal to consider yourself once before you start your detox and then after 14 days.

You may feel impatient with only two days to go! Your detox is almost over. Don't think about the detox. Instead, pamper and treat yourself. See a concert, go to a museum, get a manicure, and see a play. Anything that will distract you from what you are currently doing.

DAY 13: ALMOST DONE! WHAT DO I DO AFTER?

You may feel anxious that your detox will soon be over. You will now start planning to reintroduce some of the food that you have eliminated for this detox – beans, and dairy.

You may feel the urge to cheat since your detox is almost over. You may even call it enough since it's already day 13. Keep your goals in mind. This detox is not only about getting rid of sugar, but it's also about changing your unhealthy eating habits into a healthy one. When you make it through just one more day, the feeling of accomplishment will be awesome!

DAY 14: I MADE IT!

Sheer joy! Excitement! Pride! Relief! You pushed through and made it! Tomorrow, you can start reintroducing back the food you were not allowed to eat during the past 2 weeks.

Remember to add them back slowly to your diet.

YOUR DAILY RITUAL

Here's a reminder of what you need to do every day during your detox.

MORNING

- At the start of your day, take your measurements. Write the result in your journal – glucose, blood pressure, etc. Also, take note how many hours of sleep you got and the quality of your sleep.

- Do your 30-minute exercise – brisk walking or your preferred exercise.

- Take your PGX fiber just before breakfast.

- If taking, take your supplement with your breakfast.

- Optional: Eat your choice of mid-morning snack.

AFTERNOON

- Take your PGX fiber just before lunch.

- Enjoy your lunch.

- Optional: Eat your choice of a mid-afternoon snack.

EVENING

- Take your PGX fiber just before dinner.

- If taking, take your supplement.

- Enjoy your dinner

- Record your experience throughout the day. Jot down what you ate, what you did, how you felt, any changes and improvements in your focus and energy, and how these changes make you feel emotional, mentally, and physically. Write down any detox symptoms.

- Practice your choice of a 5-minute deep-breathing exercise.

- Sleep.

You are now ready to start your detox. Read on through the recipes and carefully plan your meal plan for two weeks. Choose from any of the following recipes or use whatever recipes are sugar detox-friendly.

CHAPTER 5: SUGAR DETOX MEAL PLAN SAMPLE

A sugar detox diet is not as complicated as you think. Just make sure that you stay clear of the foods and products that you need to avoid during the period of your detoxification. Here's a sample of what your meals will look like. It's filled with super delicious real, whole foods that are good for you.

DAY 1	
Breakfast	Spinach and Cheese Baked Eggs
Mid-Morning Snack	Toasted Tamari-Rosemary Almond
Lunch	Sweet Pepper Cheesy Poppers
Mid-Afternoon Snack	3 pieces egg, hard-boiled, remove yolk if desired
Dinner	Baked Spinach-Stuffed Chicken
DAY 2	

Breakfast	Feta and Cucumber Relish
Mid-Morning Snack	Leftover Toasted Tamari-Rosemary Almond
Lunch	Leftover Baked Spinach-Stuffed Chicken
Mid-Afternoon Snack	Cheesy Spinach Dip
Dinner	Asian-Inspired Turkey Lettuce Cups
DAY 3	
Breakfast	Peanut Butter Smoothie
Mid-Morning Snack	3 pieces egg, hard-boiled, remove yolk if desired
Lunch	Leftover Asian-Inspired Turkey Lettuce Cups with Tossed mixed green salad with tomatoes, sweet peppers, cucumber, dressed with vinegar and extra-virgin olive oil

M i d - Afternoo n Snack	Leftover Spinach and Cheese Baked Eggs
Dinner	Fresh Herb Marinated Grilled Chicken
DAY 4	
Breakfas t	Mini Frittata's
M i d - Morning Snack	1 cheese stick
Lunch	Leftover Fresh Herb Marinated Grilled Chicken with Chicken and Cilantro Salad
M i d - Afternoo n Snack	Celery dipped in sugar-free peanut butter or your preferred sugar-free nut butter
Dinner	Bean and Chicken Stew with Mini Cheesy Zucchini Bites
DAY 5	

Breakfast	Leftover Mini Frittata's
Mid-Morning Snack	Mediterranean-Inspired Spicy Feta Dip
Lunch	Leftover Bean and Chicken Stew with Tossed mixed green salad with tomatoes, sweet peppers, cucumber, dressed with vinegar and extra-virgin olive oil
Mid-Afternoon Snack	Tomato, Cucumber, and Feta Salad
Dinner	Cheesy Cauliflower Bread Sticks with Italian-Inspired Green Bean Salad
DAY 6	
Breakfast	Egg Muffin
Mid-Morning Snack	1/4 cup ricotta cheese (low fat, part-skim) tossed with a couple drops liquid vanilla stevia and 1/4 teaspoon vanilla extract

Lunch	Leftover Cheesy Cauliflower Bread Sticks with Italian-Inspired Green Bean Salad
M i d - Afternoo n Snack	Mediterranean-Inspired Spicy Feta Dip
Dinner	Lemon-Garlic Chicken Drumsticks with Zucchini Salad
DAY 7	
Breakfas t	Scrambled eggs with sautéed mushrooms and spinach with Homemade Salsa
M i d - Morning Snack	1/2 cup cottage cheese
Lunch	Vegetable Soup
M i d - Afternoo n Snack	Leftover Toasted Tamari-Rosemary Almond
Dinner	Lemon-Garlic Chicken Drumsticks with Zucchini Salad

Optional After-Dinner Snacks:

- 1/4 cup ricotta cheese (low fat, part-skim) tossed with a couple drops liquid vanilla stevia and 1/4 teaspoon vanilla extract

- 1 cheese stick

- Vanilla-Flavored Chia Pudding

- Cucumber slices topped with cottage cheese (low-fat, about ½ cup)

- 3 pieces egg, hard-boiled, remove yolk if desired

This simple sample meal plan is interchangeable, and you can adapt the recipes to your needs. If you want to customize your meal plan; feel free to search for sugar detox approved recipes and create your special one.

You may be doing this sugar detox solo and will have leftovers. You can scale down the ingredients to adjust the recipe for what you will need for the whole week.

SHOPPING LIST

Meats and Eggs	Dairy	Vegetables	Condiments or Miscellaneous
8 ounces pork sausage OR use ground turkey	8 ounces Gouda cheese, OR just use mozzarella	1 bag frozen green beans	1 jar sugar-free natural peanut butter
8 chicken drumsticks	2 packages (8-ounce each) cream cheese	1 bunch of fresh scallions or green onions	1 small-sized jar of sun-dried tomatoes
8 chicken breasts	2 cups Parmesan cheese	1 fresh head cauliflower	2 cans chicken broth, low-sodium

3 dozen eggs	2 cups feta cheese	1 pound fresh green beans	4 ounces chia seeds
1 pound ground turkey	1 package mozzarella cheese, shredded	1 pound mini sweet peppers	Fresh parsley, cilantro, and basil,
	1 package cheddar cheese, shredded	1 stalk celery	homemade hummus for snacking
	1 package cheese sticks	1 - 2 packages cherry tomatoes	homemade salsa
	1 container (16-ounce) cottage OR low-fat ricotta cheese	18 cups fresh spinach	homemade tomato sauce

	1 container (12-ounce) Greek yogurt, nonfat, plain	4 - 6 cucumbers	Low-sodium Tamari soy sauce
	1 carton unsweetened almond milk or your milk of choice	6 - 8 lemons	Powdered or liquid stevia extract
		8 fresh zucchini	Raw almonds
		8 sweet peppers, large-sized	Sesame seeds

102

		1 package (8 ounces) fresh mushrooms	Vinegar and olive oil to dress salad, also your choice of seasonings
		Frozen spinach	
		Garlic	
		Lettuce leaves for salad and Asian-Inspired Turkey Lettuce Cups	
		Onions, 2 white, and 1 red	

You can follow this meal plan or create your own. You may even know some recipes that are sugar detox-friendly. Feel free to use them.

CHAPTER 6: SUGAR DETOX RECIPES

SPINACH AND CHEESE BAKED EGGS

Serves: 6

Prep: 5 minutes

Cook: 15 minutes

Ingredients:

- 6 eggs

- 4 teaspoons olive oil, divided into 2 portions

- 2 teaspoons garlic, minced, divided into 2 portions

- 12 cups fresh spinach, divided into 2 portions

- 1 cup cheese, shredded, divided into 2 portions (I used mozzarella, low-fat)

Directions:

1. Preheat the oven to 350F.

2. Pour 2 teaspoons olive oil into a large-sized skillet.

3. Add 1 teaspoon garlic and 1/2 of the spinach. Sauté for about 2 to 3 minutes or until wilted. Add 1/2 of the cheese and then stir to combine 2 well.

4. Grease 3 ramekins with nonstick cooking spray. Divide the spinach mixture between the ramekins.

5. Cook the remaining ingredients as directed above and then divide between 3 more greased ramekins.

6. Carefully crack 1 egg over each spinach mixture.

7. Bake in the preheated oven for about 15 minutes for slightly runny yolks or bake until the desired doneness.

8. Season each serving with pepper and salt. Top with some fruit. Serve!

Toasted Tamari Almond Snack

Serves: 4

Prep: 5 minutes

Cook: 5 minutes

Ingredients:

- 2 tablespoons tamari soy sauce

- 1 cup almonds, raw

- 1 tablespoon fresh rosemary, chopped, optional

Directions:

1. Toast the raw almonds in a dry sauté pan over medium heat. Toss and cook until the almonds begin to smell delicious.

2. Remove the pan from the heat.

3. Carefully add 1 tablespoon tamari and, if using, rosemary, into the pan. Return to the burner and cook, continually stirring, until the sauce is absorbed and there are no more

juices left.

4. Let slightly chill before serving.

5. Store in an airtight container for up to 7 days.

SWEET PEPPER CHEESY POPPERS

Serves: 30

Prep: 15

Cook: 15

Ingredients:

- 1 pound mini sweet peppers, halved

- 1/2 cup feta cheese, crumbled

- 1/4 cup onion, grated

- 2 cloves garlic, minced

- 2 tablespoons cilantro, chopped

- 8 ounces cream cheese, at room temperature

- 8 ounces smoked Gouda cheese, grated

Directions:

1. Preheat the oven to425F.

2. Except for the peppers, put all of the ingredients into a bowl and mix until

combined.

3. Fill each sweet pepper half with the cheese mixture.

4. Bake in the preheated oven for 15 to 18 minutes or until the cheese is melty and slight browned.

Baked Stuffed Chicken &Spinach Recipe

Serves: 10

Prep: 10 minutes

Cook: 30 minutes

Ingredients:

- 1 cup frozen spinach, heated, excess water drained

- 1 cup marinara sauce, preferably homemade

- 1 cup ricotta cheese, part-skim

- 1 egg, beaten

- 1/2 cup mozzarella cheese, shredded

- 1/2 teaspoon salt

- 10 pieces (4 ounces) chicken breast, thin, OR 5 pieces (8-ounce) breasts, sliced into halves

- Pepper, to taste

Directions:

1. Preheat the oven to 375F.

2. Put the spinach, ricotta, egg, pepper, and salt into a mixing bowl and combine.

3. Grease a 9x13-inch baking dish with nonstick cooking spray.

4. Put the chicken breast into the greased dish. Evenly divide the spinach mixture between the chicken and put the portions on top of each breast. Roll the chicken and arrange them in the bowl with the seam side facing down.

5. Pour the marinara sauce evenly over the chicken breasts. Sprinkle all over with the mozzarella cheese.

6. Bake in the preheated oven for about 35 to 40 minutes or until the sauce is bubbling and the cheese is melted.

FETA AND CUCUMBER RELISH

Serves: 4

Prep: 10 min

Cook: 0 min

Ingredients:

- 1 cup cucumber, peeled and then chopped

- 1 cup fresh tomato, chopped

- 1 scallion, chopped

- 1 tablespoon extra-virgin olive oil

- 1/2 cup feta cheese, crumbled

- Salt and pepper, to taste

Directions:

1. Put all of the ingredients into a bowl and mix until combined.

2. Serve immediately. If not, refrigerate until ready to serve.

Feta and Sun-Dried Tomato

Frittata

Serves: 4

Prep: 5 minutes

Cook: 10 minutes

Ingredients:

- 1 clove garlic, minced

- 1/2 cup egg whites

- 1/2 cup light feta cheese, crumbled

- 1/2 cup onion, diced

- 1/2 cup sun-dried tomato, drained, chopped

- 1/4 cup almond milk, unsweetened

- 2 eggs

- 2 scallions, chopped

- 2 teaspoons coconut oil or olive oil

Directions:

1. Put the oil in a medium-sized oven-safe skillet and heat. When the oil is hot, add the onion and garlic. Sauté until the onion is translucent.

2. Add the tomatoes. Cook for about 2 to3 minutes or until heated through.

3. Meanwhile, crack the eggs, milk, and egg whites into a small-sized bowl and whisk to combine.

4. Pour the egg mixture into the skillet. Evenly sprinkle the feta cheese over the top of the egg mixture.

5. Reduce the heat to low and cook the egg mixture until the middle is almost set and the edges are set.

6. Transfer the skillet to the oven and broil for about 3 to 5 minutes or until the middle is no longer runny.

7. If desired, top with additional feta cheese and scallions.

SPINACH CHEESY

Serves: 7

Prep: 5 minutes

Cook: 5 minutes

Ingredients:

- 4 ounces Neufchatel cheese, OR lite cream cheese

- 4 cups spinach, packed into the measuring cup

- 2 teaspoons olive oil

- 1/4 teaspoon salt

- 1/4 cup Parmesan cheese

- 1 cup ricotta cheese, part-skim

- 1 clove garlic, chopped

Directions:

1. Put the oil in a sauté pan and heat. Add the garlic and spinach, Sprinkle with salt and

sauté until wilted. Set aside to cool

2. Put the Neufchatel and ricotta cheese into a blender. Blend until the mixture is smooth.

3. Add the Parmesan and cooled spinach. Pulse for 5 to 7 times or until the ingredients are incorporated – DO NOT OVER BLEND.

4. Serve immediately or refrigerate until ready to serve. Serve with your fresh raw veggies kabob– cherry tomatoes, broccoli, peppers, and cucumbers.

ASIAN TURKEY LETTUCE CUPS

Serves: 4

Prep: 15 minutes

Cook: 20 minutes

Ingredients:

- 1 carrot, large, shredded

- 1 pound ground turkey

- 1 red or yellow bell pepper, large-sized, diced

- 1 tablespoon fresh ginger, minced

- 1/2 cup mushrooms, sliced

- 1/2 cup water

- 1/2 teaspoon salt

- 1/2 teaspoon sesame seeds

- 1/4 cup fresh herbs, chopped: basil, cilantro, or mint

- 1/4 teaspoon Emeril's Asian Essence

powder

- 1/4 teaspoon garlic powder

- 1/4 teaspoon ground cinnamon

- 2 tablespoons homemade hoisin sauce

- 2 teaspoons coconut oil or olive oil

- 4 Bibb or Boston lettuce leaves, large-sized

Directions:

1. Put the oil into a large skillet and heat. Add the ginger and the turkey. Cook until the turkey is browned.

2. Add the mushrooms, pepper, hoisin sauce, and water into the skillet. Cook until heated through. Add the Asian essence, cinnamon, garlic powder, and salt. Let heat for 1 minute.

3. Wash the lettuce leaves and dry. Add 1 1/2 cups of the turkey mixture into each lettuce leaf.

4. Sprinkle the turkey mixture with the carrots, herbs, and sesame seeds.

PEANUT BUTTER SMOOTHIE

Serves: 1

Prep: 2 minutes

Cook: 0 minutes

Ingredients:

- 1/2 cup cottage cheese, low fat

- 1/2 cup almond milk, unsweetened

- 1 tablespoon peanut butter, natural, no sugar added

- 1 scoop Whey protein, optional

- 2 full droppers liquid stevia (plain, vanilla, or toffee flavor)

- 1 cup ice

Optional toppings:

- Cacao Nibs

- Peanut butter, to drizzle

Directions:

1. Put all the ingredients in a blender. Blend until the mixture is smooth.

Fresh Herb Marinated Grilled Chicken

Serves: 4

Prep: 10 minutes

Cook: 30 minutes

Ingredients:

- 1 cup mixture of fresh herbs, leaves only, loosely packed (parsley, basil, cilantro)

- 1/4 cup lemon juice

- 1/4 cup olive oil

- 1/4 teaspoon pepper

- 2 large garlic cloves

- 3 pieces (about 1 pound) chicken breasts, boneless, skinless, rinsed, patted dry, sliced lengthwise into halves

- 3 teaspoons salt

Directions:

2. Wash the herbs and then chop them. Put into a high-powered blender or food processor. Add the lemon juice, oil, pepper, salt, and garlic; process until smooth.

3. Put the chicken into a Ziploc bag. Add the marinade, seal the bag, and massage to coat the meat with the marinade. Put the container in the fridge and let marinate for at least 30 minutes and up to 8 hours.

4. When ready to serve, grill the chicken breasts for about 10-15 minutes per side or until cooked through – the meat no longer meat and the juices run clear.

VEGETABLE SOUP

Serves: 8

Prep: 10 minutes

Cook: 40 minutes

Ingredients:

- 1 cup carrots, sliced

- 1 cup green beans, frozen

- 1 cup onion, chopped

- 1/2 teaspoon garlic powder

- 1/2 teaspoon salt

- 1/4 teaspoon pepper

- 2 cloves garlic, large-sized, minced

- 2 cups celery, sliced

- 2 cups fresh spinach, chopped

- 2 cups vegetable stock or chicken broth, low sodium

- 2 teaspoons olive oil

- 4 cups water

Optional:

- 1 cup cannellini beans,

- 1 cup shelled edamame or soybeans

- 1/2 cup fresh parsley, chopped,

- Parmesan cheese, grated

Directions:

1. Put the oil into a Dutch oven and heat over medium heat. Add the garlic and sauté until fragrant.

2. Add the celery, onion, and carrots. Sauté for about 10 minutes or until the veggies are tender.

3. Pour the broth and the water into the Dutch oven and bring to a boil.

4. When boiling, add the green beans and, if using, the soybeans. Add the seasonings.

5. Cover the pot and reduce the heat to low. Simmer for 30 minutes.

6. Remove the cover. Add the parsley and spinach. Cook for about 5 minutes or until the spinach is wilted.

Vanilla-Flavored Chia Pudding

Serves: 2

Prep: 5 minutes

Cook: 0 minutes

Ingredients:

- 1/3 cup chia seeds

- 1 teaspoon vanilla extract

- 1 teaspoon liquid stevia, vanilla flavored

- 1 cup almond milk, unsweetened

- Whipped Cream, dairy-free, optional

Directions:

1. Put all the ingredients in a large pitcher and whisk until combined.

2. Divide between 2 serving glasses.

3. Refrigerate for about 10 minutes or until set.

4. If desired, top each serving with whipped

cream.

Notes: You can adjust the amount of liquid stevia. Start with 1/4 teaspoon and increase the amount to taste.

MINI FRITTATAS

Serves: 12

Prep: 10 minutes

Cook: 30 minutes

Ingredients:

- 8 ounces pork sausage

- 2 egg whites

- 2 cups yellow and red sweet peppers, diced

- 10 eggs

- 1/4 teaspoon pepper

- 1/2 teaspoon salt

- 1/2 cup pepper jack cheese

- 1/2 cup 1% milk

Optional:

- Fresh Cilantro, Chopped

- Green Onions

- Salsa, homemade

- Sour Cream, homemade

Directions:

1. Preheat the oven to 350F.

2. Cook the sausage in a skillet over medium heat until cooked through.

3. With a slotted spoon, transfer the cooked sausage to a plate and set aside.

4. In the same skillet, add the peppers and sauté until soft.

5. Crack the eggs into a large-sized bowl. Add the milk and egg whites. Whisk until combined.

6. Divide the peppers and sausage into 12 muffin cups. Pour the egg mixture into each muffin cup. Sprinkle 1 heaping tablespoon cheese over each.

7. With a fork, stir the contents of the muffin cups to combine.

8. Bake in the preheated oven for about 25 to 30 minutes.

CHICKEN AND CILANTRO SALAD

Serves: 4

Prep: 10 minutes

Cook:

Ingredients:

- 6 ounces chicken breast, cooked and chopped

- 4 yellow or red peppers, tops cut off and the insides scooped out, OR large-sized tomatoes, cut into halves, and the insides scooped out

- 1/2 cup red onion, diced

- 1/2 cup cherry tomatoes, halved

- 1 cup celery, diced

For the dressing:

- 2 tablespoons fresh cilantro, chopped

- 1/2 teaspoon salt

- 1/2 teaspoon cumin

- 1/2 cup Greek yogurt, nonfat, plain

- 1 teaspoon lemon juice

- 1 teaspoon garlic powder

- 1 tablespoon extra-virgin olive oil

Directions:

1. Put all of the dressing ingredients into a small-sized bowl and mix until combined.

2. Except for the peppers or tomatoes, put the rest of the ingredients into a large sized bowl. Add the dressing and toss to coat.

3. Put about 1 cup of the chicken salad into each tomato half or pepper.

BEAN AND CHICKEN STEW

Serves: 12

Prep: 10 minutes

Cook: 3 hours

Ingredients:

- 2 cups chicken, cooked, shredded

- 4 cups chicken broth, low-sodium

- 3 teaspoons garlic, minced

- 1/2 teaspoon salt

- 2 teaspoons cumin

- 1/2 teaspoon oregano

- 1 can hominy or corn, drained and then rinsed

- 1 can black beans, drained and then rinsed

- 1 cup salsa, homemade, OR 1 can diced tomatoes

- 1 can Lima/butter beans, Or cannellini

beans, drained and rinsed

- 1/2 cup sour cream, homemade

Optional toppings:

- Fresh cilantro

- Cheese, shredded

- Chives

- Sour cream

Directions:

1. Except for the sour cream and the optional toppings, put all of the ingredients into a crockpot. Mix to combine. Cover and cook for 3 hours on HIGH.

2. When the cooking time is up, add the sour cream to the pot and mix until well incorporated.

3. Cover the pot and cook on LOW for 30 minutes.

4. Serve topped with your preferred toppings

MINI CHEESY ZUCCHINI BITES

Serves: 3

Prep: 5 minutes

Cook: 15 minutes

Ingredients:

- 1 egg

- 1/2 cup Parmesan cheese, grated

- 1/4 cup fresh cilantro, chopped, optional

- 2 cups zucchini, grated (about 2 to 3 medium-sized)

- Salt and pepper, to taste

Directions:

1. Preheat the oven to 400F.

2. Grease a mini muffin pan with nonstick cooking spray.

3. Put the zucchini, cheese, egg, and cilantro in a bowl. Mix until combined.

4. Evenly divide the zucchini mixture between the mini muffin cups. Fill each cup to the top, patting them down if needed to pack the cups.

5. Bake for about 15 to 18 minutes or until the edges are golden brown. Check after 15 minutes.

Mediterranean-Inspired Spicy Feta Dip

Serves: 8

Prep: 10 minutes

Cook: 0 minutes

Ingredients:

- 1 cup feta cheese, reduced fat, crumbled

- 1 lemon, juice only

- 1/4 cup almond milk, unsweetened

- 1/4 cup chopped walnuts, toasted

- 1/4 cup Greek yogurt, nonfat, plain

- 1/4 cup red peppers, roasted, chopped

- 1/4 teaspoon pepper

- 1/4 teaspoon Tabasco sauce, homemade

- 2 teaspoons extra-virgin olive oil

- Kalamata or green olives, optional, for

topping

Vegetables to dip:

- Celery

- Seedless cucumbers

- Carrots

Directions:

1. Put all of the ingredients into a blender or a food processor. Pulse or blend until the mixture reaches your desired consistency.

2. Transfer to a serving bowl. If desired, top with more olives and red peppers.

3. Serve immediately or keep refrigerated until ready to serve.

CHEESY CAULIFLOWER BREAD STICKS

Serves: 4

Prep: 5 minutes

Cook: 40 minutes

Ingredients:

- 1 cup mozzarella cheese, shredded

- 1 cup Parmesan cheese, grated

- 1 teaspoon garlic powder

- 1 teaspoon Italian seasonings

- 1/2 teaspoon salt

- 2 egg whites, OR 1/4 cup egg whites

- 4 cups cauliflower, chopped (about 1 head cauliflower, washed clean and dried)

- Marinara sauce, homemade

Directions:

1. Preheat the oven to 450F.

2. Line 2 pieces of 8x12-inch baking sheets with parchment paper.

3. Microwave the cauliflower for about 7 to 8 minutes or steam for about 20 minutes or until tender.

4. Put the cooked cauliflower into a food processor; pulse until resembling rice.

5. Transfer the cauliflower rice to a large-sized bowl. Add the Parmesan cheese, seasonings, and egg whites. Mix until well combined.

6. Spread the cauliflower mixture into an even layer in one of the prepared baking sheets.

7. Put the baking sheets into the oven and bake for about 30 minutes or until the tops are browned.

8. Invert the cauliflower into the other prepared baking sheet. Put in the oven and

Bake for about 10 minutes or until the tops are browned.

9. Sprinkle the top with mozzarella cheese. Broil for about 1 minute or until the cheese is melted.

10. Let rest for 10 minutes and then slice into 24 portions.

ITALIAN-INSPIRED GREEN BEAN SALAD

Serves: 10

Prep: 5 minutes

Cook: 5 minutes

Ingredients:

- 1 1/2 pounds fresh Italian green beans, OR any kind

- 1 cup cherry tomatoes, halved

- 1/2 cup fresh basil, chopped

- 1/2 cup red onion, sliced

- 1/4 cup fresh flat or curly leaf parsley, chopped

- 2 cups English cucumber, sliced with the skin on

- 2 ounces Pecorino Romano cheese, chunks

For the Italian dressing:

- 1 lemon, juice and zest

- 1/2 teaspoon garlic powder

- 1/2 teaspoon salt

- 1/4 teaspoon pepper

- 2 tablespoons extra-virgin olive oil

- 2 tablespoons red-wine vinegar

Directions:

1. Bring a large-sized pot with water to a boil. When the water is boiling, add the beans. Blanch for 5 minutes. Immediately drain and then put the beans into an ice bath – a bowl filled with ice and water. Let fresh for about 5 to 10 minutes.

2. When the beans are chilled, drain and put into a serving bowl. Add the remaining ingredients to the pan.

3. Put all of the Italian dressing ingredients into a small-sized bowl and whisk until combined. Pour the dressing over the salad

ingredients.

4. Gently toss to coat. If needed, adjust pepper and salt to taste.

5. Serve immediately or refrigerate until ready to serve.

EGG MUFFIN

Serves: 1

Prep: 2 minutes

Cook: 2 minutes

Ingredients:

- 1 tablespoon cheese, shredded, your choice

- 1 tablespoon cream, OR milk

- 1/2 scallion, chopped

- 3 egg whites, OR 1 egg

- Nonstick cooking spray

- Salt and pepper to taste

Directions:

1. Grease a small-sized dish or a custard ramekin with nonstick cooking spray.

2. Put the egg whites/egg and cream into the dish. Whisk to combine.

3. Add the scallion and cheese. Loosely cover

the dish with a paper towel and put the plate in the microwave; microwave for about 50 to 60 seconds. If your microwave had a scrambled eggs setting, use that. Do not microwave for too long or you will have a significant mess.

Lemon-Garlic Chicken

Drumsticks

Serves: 8

Prep: 5 minutes

Cook: 20 minutes

Ingredients:

- 8 chicken drumsticks

- 3 cloves garlic, minced

- 2 tablespoons olive oil

- 2 lemons, juice only

- 1/4 cup fresh parsley, chopped

- 1/2 tablespoon butter

- 1 teaspoon salt

- 1 teaspoon pepper

- 1 teaspoon dried Italian Seasonings

- 1 lemon, zest only

Directions:

1. Put the olive oil in a large-sized sauté pan and heat.

2. While the pan is heating, season the chicken drumsticks with pepper, salt, and Italian seasoning.

3. When the oil is hot, put the chicken into the pan and cook until all the sides are browned. Transfer the drumsticks to a plate and cover with foil to keep warm.

4. Reduce the heat to low. In the same skillet, add the butter and garlic, stir for about 1 to 2 minutes. Add the lemon zest and juice. Return the drumsticks to the pan.

5. Cover and let simmer for 20 minutes.

6. Coat the drumsticks with the sauce and transfer the drumsticks to a serving plate. Pour the remaining sauce over the chicken. Garnish with chopped fresh parsley. Serve!

Zucchini Salad

Serves: 6

Prep: 10 minutes

Cook: 0 minutes

Ingredients:

- 4 zucchini, medium-sized, shredded (about 6 cups)

- 1 lemon, zest only

- 1/2 teaspoon salt

- 1/4 cup fresh parsley and basil, chopped

- 2 lemons, juice only, OR 3 tablespoons lemon juice

- 3 tablespoons extra-virgin olive oil

- Pepper, to taste

Optional toppings:

- Dried cherries

- Goat cheese

- Almonds, sliced

Directions:

1. Slice, dice, or shred the zucchini to get 6 cups total. Put into a large-sized bowl.

2. Put the oil, lemon zest and juice, pepper, and salt into a small-sized bowl and whisk until combined.

3. Pour the dressing over the zucchini. Add the parsley and basil. Gently toss to coat.

4. If desired, top with extra toppings.

5. Serve immediately or keep refrigerated until serving time.

HOMEMADE SALSA

Serves: 11

Prep: 5 minutes

Cook: 5 minutes

Ingredients:

- 1 can (28 ounces) whole peeled tomatoes, drained

- 1 cup onion, chopped

- 1 cup red pepper, chopped

- 1 tablespoon olive oil

- 1 whole jalapeno pepper, seeds and membrane removed, chopped

- 1 whole lime, juice only

- 1/2 cup fresh cilantro, chopped

- 1/2 teaspoon ground cumin

- 1/2 teaspoon salt

- 2 cans (10 ounces each) diced tomatoes with chilies

- 2 cloves garlic, chopped

Directions:

1. Put all of the ingredients into a food processor. Pulse 5 times for a chunky salsa or vibration up to 10 times for restaurant style.

2. Keep refrigerated.

FINAL WORDS

Thank you again for purchasing this book!

I really hope this book is able to help you.

The next step is for you to **join our email newsletter** to receive updates on any upcoming new book releases or promotions. You can sign-up for free and as a bonus, you will also receive our "*7 Fitness Mistakes You Don't Know You're Making*" book! This bonus book breaks down many of the most common fitness mistakes and will demystify many of the complexities and science of getting into shape. Having all this fitness knowledge and science organized into an actionable step-by-step book will help you get started in the right direction in your fitness journey! To join our free email newsletter and grab your free book, please visit the link and signup: **www.hmwpublishing.com/gift**

Finally, if you enjoyed this book, then I would like to ask you for a favor, would you be kind enough to leave a review for this book? It would be greatly appreciated!

Thank you and good luck in your journey!

About the Co-Author

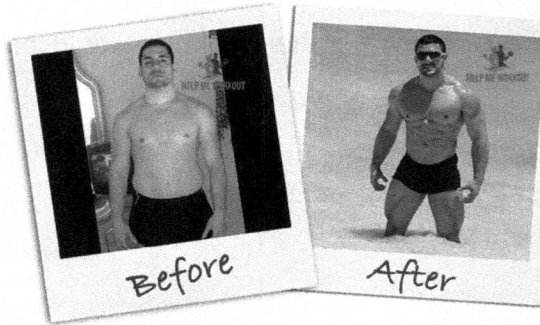

Before   After

My name is George Kaplo; I'm a certified personal trainer from Montreal, Canada. I'll start off by saying I'm not the biggest guy you will ever meet and this has never really been my goal. In fact, I started working out to overcome my biggest insecurity when I was younger, which was my self-confidence. This was due to my height measuring only 5 foot 5 inches (168cm), it pushed me down to attempt anything I ever wanted to achieve in life. You may be going through some challenges right now, or you may simply want to get fit, and I can certainly relate.

For me personally, I was always kind of interested in the health & fitness world and wanted to gain some muscle due to the numerous bullying in my teenage years about my height and my overweight body. I figured I couldn't do anything about my height, but I sure can do something about how my body looked like. This was the beginning of my transformation journey. I had no idea where to start, but I just got started. I felt worried and afraid at times that other people would make fun of me for doing the exercises the wrong way. I always wished I had a friend that was next to me who was knowledgeable enough to help me get started and "show me the ropes."

After a lot of work, studying and countless trial and errors. Some people began to notice how I was getting more fit and how I was starting to form a keen interest in the topic. This led many friends and new faces to come to me and ask me for fitness advice. At first, it seemed odd when people asked me to help them get in shape. But what kept me going is when they started to see changes in their own body and told me it's the first time that they saw real results! From there, more people kept coming to me, and it made me realize after so much reading and studying in this field that it did help me but it also allowed me to help others. I'm now a fully certified personal trainer and have trained numerous clients to date who have achieved amazing results.

Today, my brother Alex Kaplo (also a Certified Personal Trainer) and I own & operate this publishing venture, where we bring passionate and expert authors to write about health and fitness topics. We also run an online fitness website "HelpMeWorkout.com" and I would love to connect with by inviting you to visit the website on the following page and signing up to our e-mail newsletter (you will even get a free book).

Last but not least, if you are in the position I was once in and you want some guidance, don't hesitate and ask... I'll be there to help you out!

Your friend and coach,

George Kaplo

Certified Personal Trainer

Download another book for

Free

I want to thank you for purchasing this book and offer you another book (just as long and valuable as this book), "Health & Fitness Mistakes You Don't Know You're Making", completely free.

Visit the link below to signup and receive it:

www.hmwpublishing.com/gift

In this book, I will break down the most common health & fitness mistakes, you are probably committing right now, and I will reveal how you can easily get in the best shape of your life!

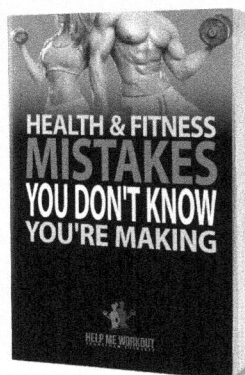

In addition to this valuable gift, you will also have an opportunity to get our new books for free, enter giveaways, and receive other valuable emails from me. Again, visit the link to sign up:

www.hmwpublishing.com/gift

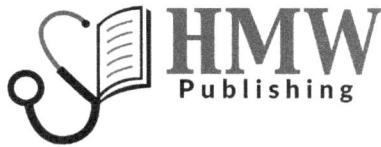

For more great books visit:

HMWPublishing.com

www.ingramcontent.com/pod-product-compliance
Lightning Source LLC
Chambersburg PA
CBHW060310030426
42336CB00011B/990